Intellectual Disabilities *and* Dual Diagnosis

An Interprofessional Clinical Guide for Healthcare Providers

Bruce D. McCreary and Jessica Jones

Queen's Policy Studies Series
School of Policy Studies, Queen's University
McGill-Queen's University Press
Montreal & Kingston • London • Ithaca

Queen's University

SCHOOL OF
Policy Studies

Publications Unit
Robert Sutherland Hall
138 Union Street
Kingston, ON, Canada
K7L 3N6
www.queensu.ca/sps/

Library and Archives Canada Cataloguing in Publication

McCreary, Bruce D.
[Developmental disabilities and dual diagnosis]
Intellectual disabilities and dual diagnosis : an interprofessional clinical guide for healthcare providers / Bruce D. McCreary and Jessica Jones.

(Queen's policy studies series)
Revision of author's Developmental disabilities and dual diagnosis.
Includes bibliographical references and index.
Issued in print and electronic formats.
ISBN 978-1-55339-331-3 (pbk.). ISBN 978-1-55339-337-5 (ebook).
ISBN 978-1-55339-340-5 (pdf).

1. People with mental disabilities—Medical care—Handbooks, manuals, etc.
2. People with mental disabilities—Diseases—Handbooks, manuals, etc.
3. Developmentally disabled—Medical care—Handbooks, manuals, etc.
4. Developmentally disabled—Diseases—Handbooks, manuals, etc. 5. Mental retardation—Handbooks, manuals, etc. 6. Medical personnel—Handbooks, manuals, etc.
I. Jones, Jessica, 1971- II. Title. III. Series: Queen's policy studies series

RC570.M36 2013 362.2 C2013-904065-X
C2013-906760-4

CONTENTS

FOREWORD

Few areas of clinical practice are as potentially complex and demanding as those covered in this book. This term *intellectual disabilities* encompasses an extremely heterogeneous group of people who not only vary in their personalities and their cultural and family backgrounds, as do we all, but also in the extent, nature, and cause of their disability. This complexity is compounded by high rates of physical and psychiatric comorbidities and by specific maladaptive behaviours that impact negatively on individuals and families. *Intellectual Disabilities and Dual Diagnosis: An Interprofessional Clinical Guide for Healthcare Providers* helps make sense of this and provides a solid and conceptually sound framework for assessment and intervention. The book moves logically from a focus on the person's intellectual disability itself, through physical and mental health problems, to an account of the skills and services required, to finally a reflection on the attitudes that health professionals need toward the person with an intellectual disability and their family, as well as toward providers in other disciplines.

What then are some of the key themes identified in this guide? First, as described above, there is the theme of complexity. It is for this reason that what is required in the support of someone with an intellectual disability and a dual diagnosis is a structured process of information gathering, which then leads to the development of a formulation. This formulation brings together what is known about the individual and his/her surroundings, and information based on the most appropriate and theoretically sound conceptual models of understanding, to inform intervention.

The second theme is interdisciplinary and interagency collaboration. Again, as clearly set out the book, a range of knowledge and skills is needed to arrive at an understanding and to ultimately inform and deliver a particular intervention or interventions. Healthcare professionals may have to gather the history of a person's difficulties through a third party, and the interventions may be delivered by family members or by those paid to provide social support. This interface between health and social care can be problematic, as different perspectives and cultures may collide.

A third theme is the developmental perspective that must inform our understanding of the delayed or atypical developmental trajectories of those being supported and also how, over a lifetime, needs change as do which organizations meet these needs. As a person with an intellectual disability ages, the focus will shift from an initial diagnostic one, "Why isn't my child developing normally?", to developing educational and functional skills at school, to moving toward greater independence in adolescence and adult life, developing appropriate support strategies, and addressing issues around sexuality or emerging age-related comorbidities such as mood disorders. The co-occurrence in one person of an intellectual disability and autistic spectrum disorder is one example of how identifying a particular developmental trajectory can inform intervention. Similarly, increasing knowledge about the particular physical and mental health risks associated with specific genetically determined neurodevelopmental syndromes informs clinical practice and also research—often now referred to as the "behavioural phenotype" of that syndrome. For example, knowing about the biologically determined failure of satiety in people with Prader-Willi Syndrome and the associated overeating behaviour and risk of life-threatening obesity is central to the development of support strategies. There are an increasing number of such examples in those with other genetically determined neurodevelopmental syndromes.

The final theme that this guide covers fits well with the section on attitudes but is perhaps wider than that. It encompasses legal and ethical aspects of the support of people with intellectual disabilities and the treatment of comorbidity. Tensions may arise between interventions designed to prevent or treat ill-health on the one hand, and the wish to support people to be independent and to make their own choices on the other. While these aims should not be in opposition, they may be, and their resolution may crucially depend on the attitudes of all those involved. For example, someone may refuse consent to an invasive investigation or an unpleasant but potentially life-saving treatment, perhaps through fear. People with intellectual disabilities may not understand why they are in pain, that their lives are at risk, and that treatment will ameliorate the problem. How, in such circumstances, should healthcare professionals balance what may be competing rights—the right to self-determination and the right to life? These issues are addressed through legislation at the national level, but often decisions have to be made in circumstances that are far from easy and where there may be disagreements as to the best approach. There are also the wider concerns about risk and protection from harm that come under the umbrella of "safeguarding." How to recognize possible abuse and how to respond?

This book is an invaluable source to help you collect and structure the necessary information in these often complex situations and to make decisions that are clinically, ethically, and legally justifiable. No book can tell you exactly what to do in any given situation—that requires skilled judgment. However, a guide such as this can provide a structured approach that helps bring order to what at times may be a confusing and even chaotic situation. I congratulate the authors on the work they have done.

Anthony Holland
Cambridge Intellectual and Developmental Disabilities Research Group
Department of Psychiatry, University of Cambridge, United Kingdom
October 2013

Preface

Significant mental impairments that start early in life and tend to persist are often called "developmental disabilities." A person with a developmental disability complicated by another mental disorder has a "dual diagnosis." These mental impairments distort and delay the person's maturation and personal growth, preventing success in developmental, educational, and vocational endeavours.

This guide illustrates the interprofessional challenges involved in the care of persons with developmental disabilities and dual diagnosis. We have chosen to deemphasize some of the controversies involved in the definition and categorization of various developmental disabilities, and to focus instead on the significant challenges involved in ensuring optimal care for those affected and support for their caregivers.

Individuals with a developmental disability (e.g., an intellectual disability) or with a dual diagnosis are high on the list of those who experience healthcare disparities. They are in a disadvantaged position in relation to other citizens, owing to an unfortunate combination of complex healthcare needs and poor training of healthcare professionals to address those needs. Similar considerations apply to the provision of education and social services.

Given there are no short-term solutions to preventing the unique "special needs" of persons with developmental disabilities, efforts to improve professional training are critically important. Presently, most jurisdictions (certainly Canada is among them) have yet to ensure adequate training about developmental disabilities. With respect to healthcare, for example, people with developmental disabilities suffer from the same illnesses as members of the general population, but they have more illnesses at once, and frequently rely on caregivers to manage these complex comorbidities. They are not "average" healthcare consumers. It is therefore essential that healthcare professionals understand how the needs of people with developmental disabilities differ from the majority, and how to assist them. These issues must be addressed in training programs, both for primary caregivers and for specialists.

An earlier version of this guide, *Developmental Disabilities and Dual Diagnosis: A Guide for Canadian Psychiatrists,* was published in 2005. Although written primarily for psychiatrists-in-training, that guide has been widely used to train other healthcare professionals. Many already in practice, whose training in the field of developmental disabilities had been inadequate, also found it to be a helpful resource. Accordingly, in preparing a new edition, we have endeavoured to accommodate the interprofessional learning needs of all healthcare professionals-in-training as well as the interests of those already in practice. Most sections have been updated and rewritten to include new advances in interprofessional collaborative care and education.

We acknowledge the support of our colleagues in the Division of Developmental Disabilities in the Department of Psychiatry, Queen's University. We also thank our clients and their caregivers who are our best teachers about developmental disabilities and dual diagnosis.

How to Use This Guide

Establishing relationships with people who have developmental disabilities can be a challenge. Their characteristic cognitive and communication impairments, often associated with fear in novel situations, represent important barriers to receiving help from healthcare professionals.

Because individuals with developmental disabilities are predisposed to various health and mental health problems, an uncertain relationship with a healthcare provider is particularly worrisome. In these circumstances providers need optimal levels of knowledge and clinical skills, not to mention empathetic attitudes to ensure productive encounters. Topics that need to be addressed include how to

- collect comprehensive clinical histories,
- interview and examine reluctant and anxious individuals,
- obtain "informed consent" for treatment, and
- communicate treatment recommendations to caregivers.

This guide focuses on the provision of interprofessional healthcare services for persons with developmental disabilities. It assumes that readers need to learn about the nature and causes of developmental disabilities, the educational and social services required, the predisposing health and mental health problems, and the skills and attitudes involved in providing quality care.

The guide uses a clinical handbook approach to presentation and content. It is organized into three parts: knowledge, skills, and attitudes. Within each part are five subsections with targeted learning objectives. Each subsection summarizes key issues and suggests further readings for those who want to learn more. Appendices provide formats for

- recording clinical histories,
- formulating comprehensive management/treatment plans, and
- "self-testing" on the guide's contents.

Case vignettes illustrating common clinical scenarios provide opportunities for readers to conceptualize and plan interventions.

Readers need to understand the importance of supervised practicum experiences in learning about developmental disabilities. Neither this guide nor traditional textbooks can alone promote the acquisition of optimal skills and attitudes that occurs in clinical settings.

Although the guide includes a glossary, a few words on terminology are needed. The terms used to refer to persons with developmental disabilities vary across jurisdictions and over time within jurisdictions. These shifts often reflect the stigma that becomes attached to terms over time. Each "new" term has a life cycle of 15–20 years and is inevitably replaced. "Developmental disabilities" is the term currently in use in North America to refer to the diagnosis of mental retardation and pervasive developmental disabilities as defined by the American Psychiatric Association manual. "Learning disabilities" is widely used as an alternative in the United Kingdom.

More generally, the term "intellectual disabilities" is emerging as a preferable option internationally. "Dual diagnosis" is commonly used to refer to persons with both an intellectual disability and mental health problem, but this term in not found in any officially sanctioned nosologies.

BRUCE D. MCCREARY
JESSICA JONES

FURTHER READINGS:

American Psychiatric Association. (2000). *Diagnostic and statistical manual of mental disorders* (4th ed.). Arlington, VT: Author.

Pasquale, J. A., & Whitman, B. Y. (2011). *Dictionary of developmental disabilities terminology* (3rd ed.). Baltimore: Paul H. Brookes.

Part 1 – Knowledge

Individuals with developmental disabilities and dual diagnosis need the assistance of a wide variety of professionals over their lifetime. To treat and support these individuals, healthcare professionals need two sets of knowledge: core and supplementary. The core knowledge is based on awareness of the adaptive problems that result from early-onset cognitive impairment, and on related health and mental health comorbidities. This knowledge informs the professional skills required for assessment, diagnosis, and treatment. Healthcare professionals must also learn how to advocate effectively within the health, education, developmental, and social service sectors. In addition to core knowledge, therefore, supplementary knowledge about cross-sectoral and interministerial relationships is necessary for success.

The core and supplementary knowledge is recorded in a broad range of professional sources. While some is found in mainstream publications, often it has been placed in international specialty journals like the *American Journal on Intellectual and Developmental Disabilities* or the UK *Journal of Intellectual Disability Research*. The journal *Current Opinion in Psychiatry* provides an annual review designed to summarize important advances in the field gleaned from multiple primary sources.

Books and monographs providing more extensive coverage of health and mental health problems in developmental disabilities will also be of interest; three are recommended here.

Bouras, N., & Holt, G. (Eds.). (2010). *Mental health services for adults with intellectual disability: Strategies and solutions*. London: Routledge and Psychology Press.

O'Brien, G., & Rosenbloom, L. (2010). *Developmental disability and aging*. London: Mackeith Press.

O'Hara, J., McCarthy, J., & Bouras, N. (2010). *Intellectual disability and ill health: A review of the evidence*. Cambridge: Cambridge University Press.

1.1 To understand the impact of different levels of intellectual impairment on an individual's adaptive behaviour in childhood and at maturity

Knowledge of the impact of different levels of intellectual impairment on the adaptive potential of persons with developmental disabilities is a key consideration for healthcare professionals in serving this population. This knowledge not only provides the basis for the formulation of a treatment-management plan for each individual who is referred but also shapes the clinician's approach to assessment of the presenting problems.

In the general population, "normal" mental development means that each young person will demonstrate competence in attaining basic daily living skills (e.g., self-help, communication with others) and in education. At maturity, each adult is expected to have employment and family responsibilities. For individuals with developmental disabilities, the normal pattern of development is disrupted or distorted. Because the genetic and environmental insults that cause developmental disabilities vary in severity, there are different levels of intellectual impairment from mild to profound. While the level of intellectual functioning can be estimated clinically from an interview, a developmental history, and a mental status examination (see Section 2.1), more precise testing with standardized psychometric tools like the Stanford-Binet Intelligence Scales or the Wechsler Adult Intelligence Scales is usually undertaken. Intelligence Quotients (IQs) are used to categorize the level of intellectual disability as follows:

Level of Intellectual Disability	*IQ Range*
Mild	50–55 to 70
Moderate	35–40 to 50–55
Severe	20–25 to 35–40
Profound	less than 20–25

The level of intellectual disability is considered "unspecified" when psychometric test results are not available or assessment has been deemed not valid or interpretable.

Levels of adaptive behaviour, like levels of intellectual impairment, can also be assessed clinically or by use of standardized measures such as the Vineland Adaptive Behaviour Scale. These measures typically list the following categories of adaptive behaviour: self-care, communication, home living, social/interpersonal skills, self-direction, functional academic skills, work, leisure, health, and safety.

Formal definition of a diagnosis of "mental retardation" in standard nosologies includes subaverage intellectual functioning, impaired adaptive behaviour, and onset prior to age 18 years.

Family members, teachers, social workers, and other caregivers often want to know what levels of functional ability and academic competency they might expect for the individual in the near and distant future. To answer these questions, clinicians need to consider variables apart from intellectual level, such as the effects of comorbid disabilities, motivational factors, and environmental opportunities for learning for the individual. Table 1 illustrates levels of intellectual impairment and competence for progressive life stages. Various comorbid disabilities are described in subsequent sections, but for now it should be observed that these tend to cluster in those with increasingly severe levels of intellectual impairment.

An implication for clinicians in preparing case formulations for persons with developmental disabilities is the so-called inverse care law: people with high levels of need tend to get lower levels of treatment and care. In other words, "The less you have, the less you get." Special attention is needed to accommodate multiple cognitive and physical impairments in those with a cluster of comorbidities, particularly if the individual has also experienced marginalization or neglect with resultant demoralization or helplessness.

Clinicians should be aware of clinical outliers such as individuals who present with significant problems in adaptive behaviour but whose intelligence scores are above the range used to define intellectual disability or "mental retardation." Clinically, some young children are identified as "developmentally delayed" because they are behind expectations in achieving their developmental milestones. But when they are tested at age 3–4, their IQ scores are not found to be "significantly subaverage," and so the term "mental retardation" is not applied.

Many individuals with autism spectrum disorder have intellectual functioning in the borderline range (IQ of 70–85), a level previously classified as "borderline mental retardation." These individuals are sometimes identified by schools and social agencies as having mild intellectual impairment. However, their adaptive behaviour is likely to be compromised more by social difficulties in relating to others and by obsessional behaviours than by intellectual impairment alone.

Many assume that a diagnosis of mental retardation is permanent. However, children diagnosed with a mild developmental disability sometimes, as adults, successfully manage vocational and family responsibilities without external supports. When this occurs, their needs may no longer meet the adaptive behaviour requirement of the diagnosis. This pattern explains changes in the administrative prevalence of developmental disability; that is, in the number of cases receiving service in a given population at a specific point in time. The peak administrative prevalence of developmental disability is 3% at approximately age 12 when adaptation in school is invariably problematic. By adulthood, it has dropped to 1% when many of those with mild intellectual impairment have learned to adapt successfully in employment and family life.

TABLE 1
Outline of Competencies in Persons with Mental Retardation

Level of Intellectual Impairment	*Levels of Competence*		
	Preschool Years	*School Years*	*Adulthood*
Mild	Normal developmental landmarks* apart from possible delays in language and communication skills.	Development of literacy and numeracy skills. Academic achievement to around Grade 6 level.	Maintains manual or unskilled employment. May need income support to promote independence. Often develops stable relationships. Parenting skills are possible with support.
Moderate	Frequent developmental delays especially in speech and language.	Focus on communication and social skills. Academic achievement to around Grade 2.	Obtains supported employment, and needs income support. May require regular residential supervision, and support with banking and shopping. Usually does not have the understanding and competence to be a parent.
Severe	Significant delays in cognitive, sensorimotor, speech, and language skills.	Focus on functional needs and specific support in self-care, language, and communication skills.	Needs regular support and supervision in residential care and daycare programs. Unable to manage "family" responsibilities.
Profound	Major delays in cognitive, sensorimotor, speech, and language skills.	Requires 24-hour support and supervision. Focus on self and communication skills.	Needs continuing 24-hour support and supervision. Unable to manage "family" responsibilities.

Notes: * Developmental landmarks: smiles at mother, 4–6 weeks; sits unsupported, 7–8 months; walks, 12–14 months; speaks individual words, 12 months; joins words together, 24 months; dry during the day, 2 years; dry at night, 3 years.

Further Readings:

American Psychiatric Association. (2000). *Desk reference to diagnostic criteria from DSM-IV-TR.* Washington, DC: Author.

Gottfredson, L. S. (1998). The general intelligence factor. *Scientific American, 9*(4), 24-29.

Illingworth, R. S. (1975). *The development of the infant and young child: Normal and abnormal* (6th ed.). Edinburgh: Churchill-Livingston.

Miller, A. R. (1994). Developmental delay recognition, evaluation and subsequent action. *Canadian Journal of Paediatrics, 1*(4), 145-151.

O'Brien, G. (2001). Adult outcome of childhood learning disability. *Developmental Medicine & Child Neurology, 43*(9), 634-638.

1.2 To understand the contribution of genetic factors and environmental influences to the etiology of developmental disabilities and dual diagnosis

Our current understanding of the causes of developmental disabilities and dual diagnosis is based on observations made by a wide variety of scientists and clinicians over many years, and advances are made on a continuing basis. Although practitioners are not expected to be well versed on each and every cause, they must be familiar with the range of etiological possibilities and know where to refer for definitive answers. Family members and agency caregivers are keenly interested in causes and gaining further understanding, even when this knowledge does not appear to affect immediate care.

An approach to establishing and understanding the causes of "mental defect" (i.e., intellectual disability and any comorbid mental disorder) was pioneered by the late Lionel Penrose. He pointed out that major genetic and environmental insults to mental development must be considered in relation to "normal variation" observed in population studies of intelligence. While normal variation involves the interplay of multiple genetic and environmental influences, extremes in mental status often follow single "pathological" genetic mutations or biomedical insults that seriously interfere with normal brain growth and development.

Most individuals with mild intellectual impairment fall within the lower range of normal variation. Although the number and identity of individual genes that are involved has not been determined, collectively they account for approximately 50% of the variability. The other 50% relates to a variety of biomedical and psychosocial factors that determine brain function and mental development. Persons with mild intellectual impairment appear to have experienced a larger share of deterrents to normal intellectual development such as poor maternal health during pregnancy, poor nutrition during childhood, and inadequate sensory and language stimulation. These kinds of deterrents are more commonly found in lower socioeconomic groups, which accounts for the observed associations between social disadvantage and mild intellectual impairment. Presently, increasing attention is given to reducing health and social inequities during the formative years so that those with mild intellectual impairment can adapt successfully as adults in assuming meaningful vocational and family responsibilities. This approach is in marked contrast to the early years of the last century when a societal preoccupation with eugenics promoted segregation of the sexes and involuntary sterilization.

Individuals with moderate, severe, and profound levels of intellectual impairment owe the majority of their difficulties, as already noted, to pathological factors that seriously disrupt the development and function of the central nervous system. These individuals are represented in all socioeconomic levels in society and are more likely than persons with mild intellectual impairment to suffer from comorbidities such as epilepsy and cerebral palsy.

These comorbidities are usually linked to the same neuropathology that causes the intellectual impairment. Occasionally, the pathological category also describes individuals with mild intellectual disabilities, an indication of the inevitable overlap between pathological and normal variation.

Given a list of at least 200 disorders that can cause significant intellectual impairment, most clinicians can only endeavour to have a conceptual framework for categorizing etiologies, as shown in Figure 1. In addition, clinicians need an approach to each individual that allows for systematic analysis of rare, or even unique, circumstances.

FIGURE 1
A Developmental Framework That Accommodates Genetic, Environmental, and Idiopathic Disorders

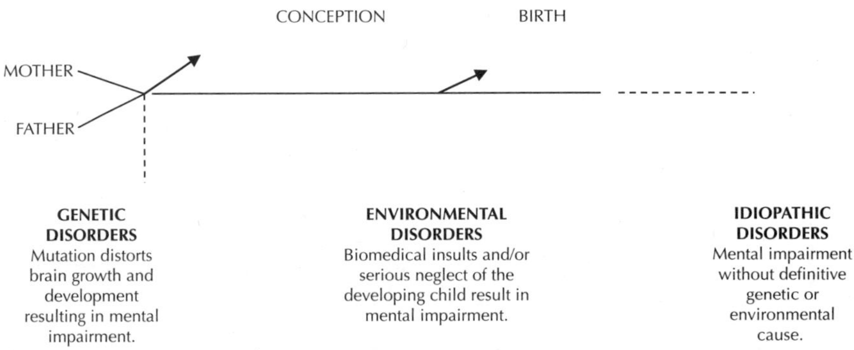

In this framework, particular disorders are listed under one of the three main headings. Genetic disorders can be subdivided into various categories such as Down syndrome (a chromosomal disorder), Fragile X (a tri nucleotide repeat disorder), and tuberous sclerosis (a single gene disorder). Using birth as a dividing point, environmental disorders can be subdivided as well, for example, into fetal alcohol abuse syndrome (prenatal), asphyxia at birth (perinatal), and post meningitic intellectual disability (postnatal). And finally, idiopathic cases can be subcategorized to facilitate further etiological analysis, such as those with or without comorbid epilepsy or congenital anomalies.

In keeping with the Penrose approach, considerable clinical effort is expended on identifying "syndromes" so that further study of particular disorders will help to delineate specific methods of treatment or prevention. Perhaps the best example of this evolution in the understanding of a particular disorder is phenylketonuria, a metabolic disorder inherited recessively, whose damaging effects can be prevented by adhering to a diet low in phenylalanine. Given advances in describing "behavioural phenotypes" associated with syndromes (i.e., behavioural characteristics of different genetic disorders), mental health professionals can usefully contribute to these important areas of research.

With respect to comorbid psychiatric illnesses, like schizophrenia or bipolar illness, it seems clear that etiological considerations relevant in the general population apply to those with developmental disabilities. However, research has revealed some interesting predispositions in persons with particular syndromes; for example, persons with Down syndrome are predisposed to Alzheimer's disease, and those with velocardiofacial syndrome to psychosis. In these examples, genes that are presumed to be critical in the pathogenesis of the mental disorder are linked to the chromosome abnormalities observed in the syndrome.

A clinical approach that can be used to define syndromes and placement in an etiological category is described in Section 2.1. Assessment should occur as early as possible in the individual's life and need only be repeated if there are unexpected recurrences in the family or new scientific evidence that raises the possibility of improved definition of cases previously labelled "idiopathic."

Parents and other family members are naturally inquisitive about the causes of cognitive impairment and frequently ask clinicians about the matter even when apprehensive about the possible answer. If they do not inquire, at some juncture a clinician should initiate discussions about what is presently known, pointing out that some time in the future research may explain a case that is currently idiopathic. If a genetic assessment of the immediate family has not yet been completed, the clinician should discuss the value and possible implications with family members. Any obvious misunderstandings about common concerns such as the impact of "birth injury" or emotional shock during pregnancy should be corrected.

Further Readings:

Abel, E. L. (1998). *Fetal alcohol abuse syndrome.* New York: Plenum Press.

Centerwall, S. A., & Centerwall, W. R. (2000). The discovery of phenylketonuria: The story of a young couple, two retarded children and a scientist. *Pediatrics, 105*, 85-104.

Firth, H. V., Hurst, J. A., & Hall, J. G. (2005). *Oxford desk reference: Clinical genetics.* Oxford: Oxford University Press.

O'Brien, G., & Yule, W. (Eds.). (1995). *Behavioural phenotypes.* Cambridge: Cambridge University Press.

Penrose, L. S. (1963). *The biology of mental defect.* London: Sidgwich and Jackson.

1.3 To understand the role of developmental programs, case management, and social services in providing care and support for persons with intellectual disabilities and dual diagnosis, and their families

Knowledge about the various developmental, educational, and social services needed over the lifetime of persons with developmental disabilities and their families is "supplementary" knowledge for healthcare providers. Its relevance relates to a number of practical issues encountered in providing care, such as predicting levels of competency, identifying the personal impact of gaps in support services, and evaluating adjustment disorders arising from problematic relationships between individuals and support agencies.

Care for persons with developmental disabilities and their families involves a broad range of services and professionals beyond the healthcare sector. While healthcare providers can be expected to be fully acquainted with health services, the same level of knowledge about developmental, educational, and social services is impossible. Yet clinicians will likely encounter a number of important non-health issues in the course of normal practice. Is the student with a disability not meeting expected levels of competence because of inadequate resources or problematic relationships in the school? Is the family breaking down because they have not received the special financial allowance to which they are entitled? Such issues reflect legitimate and important concerns for individuals with disabilities and their families. These issues are comparable to the effects of financial, social, and personal stressors on the health of the general population, although among those with disabilities the impacts will likely be more complex.

In these circumstances, it can be very useful for clinicians to refer to a model of care and support that reflects the evolving needs of individuals with disabilities and their families (Figure 2). Such a model can help clinicians to address practical issues.

The model is "developmental" inasmuch as the complete interval between birth and death is subdivided into three successive stages: childhood, maturity, and senescence. With the three model elements—developmental programs, case management, and social services—a matrix is created, including two critical stages for planning: transition (between childhood and maturity) and permanency (following the inevitable death of the parents).

Developmental programs aim to maximize and maintain the adaptive capacities of the person with a disability over the lifespan. During childhood, these programs focus on early intervention and education. "Productivity" at maturity includes any teaching or retraining that will assist the person in contributing to his or her own welfare through relevant life skills or employment. And during senescence, "activity" is concerned with life skills that enhance quality of life in the person's later years.

FIGURE 2
A Model of Care and Support for Persons With Intellectual Disability

MODEL ELEMENTS	BIRTH CHILDHOOD		DEVELOPMENT → → MATURITY		DEATH SENESCENCE
Developmental Programs	Early Intervention and Education	TRANSITION PLANNING	Productivity/ Employment	PERMANENCY PLANNING	Activity
Case Management	Recognition & Case Register		Case Coordination		Case Coordination
Social Services	Family Services		Personal Support		Old Age Security

Case management ensures coordination of services on behalf of the individual with a disability and the family. It can include facilitating professional assessments of the individual's mental and physical impairments, convening interprofessional case conferences, and developing and monitoring management plans. Case managers also provide advice to families about navigating the complexities of the healthcare, education, and social service sectors. Transition and permanency planning are focused on critical junctures during the lifespan when major adjustments are needed. Moving from school to the workplace or from reliance on parents to reliance on other caregivers requires anticipatory case management if unnecessary stress and possible decompensation are to be avoided. Although case registers are not widely available in North America, they can be a uniquely valuable resource in forecasting caseloads that will be faced by agencies and professionals serving a defined geographic area (see Section 3.3).

Finally, professionals in *social services* seek to maintain personal and family resources relevant to living with chronic/persistent adaptive problems and to ensure quality of life for those involved. "Family services" represents supports for parents of a child with a disability and can include counselling, respite care, and financial allowances. When the person reaches maturity, social services assist with housing, residential supervision, day programs, and income support. These services continue as Old Age Security during senescence.

During the last 25 years of the 20th century, there was a major shift in public policy with respect to persons with developmental disabilities.

Advocates dissatisfied with the care provided in institutions, and further dissatisfied with an almost complete absence of community-based supports, lobbied strongly for a policy on deinstitutionalization. This policy, widely accepted in developed countries around the world, meant that admissions to institutions were stopped, that those living in institutions were relocated to the community, and that schools and social agencies integrated persons with developmental disabilities into their mainstream programs. Unfortunately, the challenges faced by communities and the "social cost" of the new social inclusion policy have been underestimated. In practice, this means that clinicians will encounter individuals who, although living in the community, are socially isolated, unoccupied, and unhappy—primarily because of shortcomings in the level of support they receive. In spite of these problems, policy statements for the 21st century never mention a return to institutional care but stress goals like rights, independence, choice, and inclusion in the community. In setting such goals, policy-makers often underestimate the need for enhanced resources.

Persons with developmental disabilities have wide variations in their needs and aspirations. The creation of a reliable and valid tool to assess support needs and associated resources has therefore been a major challenge. The Supports Intensity Scale (SIS), currently utilized in North America, is an important innovation. The SIS is a structured interview, administered by a trained assessor, with two or more informants who know the individual with a disability well. It evaluates 57 "life" activities, 16 "exceptional" medical needs, and 13 "behavioural support" needs. It is used in several states and provinces to develop individual support plans and to allocate funding arrangements for adults with developmental disabilities living in the community.

Further Readings:

Odom, S., Horner, R. H., Snell, M. E., & Blacher, J. (2007). *Handbook of developmental disabilities.* New York: Guilford Press.

Wehmeyer, M., Chapman, T., & Little, T. (2009). Efficacy of the Supports Intensity Scale (SIS) to predict extraordinary support needs. *American Journal of Intellectual and Developmental Disabilities, 114*(1), 3-14.

1.4 To understand the comorbid health problems that influence the adjustment and quality of life of persons with developmental disabilities

Individuals with developmental disabilities are susceptible to the same health problems experienced by members of the general population. They are also predisposed to certain health problems, some reviewed in this section, that can present behaviourally or otherwise contribute to the pathogenesis of mental health problems. In either case, clinicians concerned about dual diagnosis need to understand these important associations between health and mental health problems. Clinicians in mainstream health services cannot avoid these associations, particularly the possibility that a change in behaviour, reported by a caregiver of someone with significant communication difficulties, is a signal that medical or dental treatment is urgently required.

Surveys of morbidity and mortality rates for persons with developmental disabilities over the past 30 years have already indicated the importance of monitoring their health status (e.g., with annual health checks) and of creating special linkages between primary caregivers and hospitals (e.g., with "hospital passports") to ensure prompt interventions when a serious illness occurs.

Further Readings:

Michael, J. (Sir). (2008). *Health care for all: Report of the independent inquiry into access to healthcare for people with learning disabilities.* Chiswick: Aldridge Press.

Sullivan, W. E., Berg, J. M., & Bradley, E., Cheetham, T., Denton, R. Heng, J. ... McMillan, S. (2011). Primary care of adults with developmental disabilities: Canadian consensus guidelines. *Canadian Family Physician, 57*(5), 541-553.

1.4.1 Congenital Anomalies

Congenital anomalies (i.e., physical abnormalities present from birth) are prevalent in persons with developmental disabilities. Their presence reflects the impact of genetic or environmental insults to normal embryonic development. Anomalous development of the brain causes functional problems that create additional adaptive challenges. "Major" congenital malformations (e.g., cleft lip and palate, defects of the heart and great vessels) usually require surgical correction and, even then, can be associated with premature mortality. "Minor" congenital anomalies, like fusion of the second and third toes, cause little if any functional impairment and have no effect whatsoever on longevity.

Surgical management of major congenital anomalies is extremely stressful for the person with disabilities and the family. Frequent or extended stays in hospital, uncertainty about outcome, and high risk of premature death can disrupt parent-child attachment and bonding. Attachment problems are a significant risk, even though children's hospitals do everything possible to prevent these risks.

Neural tube defects (anencephaly, hydrocephalus, and spina bifida) deserve special mention. Anencephaly is associated with stillbirth or early neonatal death. Unless spontaneous arrest of progressive hydrocephalus occurs, cerebrospinal fluid shunts are needed; the clinician may be presented with complaints of headache or a personality change in an older individual whose shunt has blocked and needs surgical revision. Spina bifida varies in severity but many have paralyzed lower limbs, incontinence, and recurrent urinary tract infections with obvious impacts on adaptive behaviour and quality of life.

Mental health consultation is often requested when an individual who has multiple congenital anomalies also experiences mood difficulties, low frustration tolerance, and interpersonal difficulties with family or agency caregivers.

Minor congenital anomalies in isolation may have little functional significance but when clustered together can cause health problems. In Down syndrome, for example, a narrowed airway, large tongue, and muscle hypotonia predispose sleep apnea; this condition must be considered in the differential diagnosis of daytime somnolence, depression, and dementia. Abnormalities of sensory organs are usually associated with abnormal hearing or vision, a topic considered further in Section 1.4.2, given the obviously important adaptive limitations that occur. Problems with mastication, swallowing, and speech and language development are associated with anomalous development of the maxilla and mandible.

Further Reading:

Caplan, L. C. (1989). Assessment and management of infants and children with multiple congenital anomalies. In I. L. Rubin & A. C. Crocker (Eds.), *Developmental disabilities: Delivery of medical care for children and adults* (pp. 97-116). Philadelphia: Lea and Febiger Publishers.

1.4.2 Sensory Impairments

Vision and hearing impairments in persons with developmental disabilities may be caused by congenital abnormalities of the sensory organs or acquired through infection, trauma, or degenerative disorders as seen in the general population. Regardless of their origin, sensory impairments create additional adaptive challenges beyond the individual's primary cognitive limitations.

Childhood-onset hearing and vision impairments are associated with "developmental delay," and evaluation of at-risk children must include appropriate sensory screening. Child development experts, given the heterogeneity of the population with developmental delays and uncertainty about how to best measure intelligence in children with sensory impairments, often disagree about how much of the cognitive limitation can be ascribed to sensory problems. There is a consensus, however, that incidental learning is reduced and that atypical developmental trajectories occur. Children who have hearing impairments or deafness have been found to have short attention spans and are often described as restless or "fidgety." Children who are visually impaired or blind are found to be hypotonic and can be inclined to engage in stereotypic behaviours. Both groups present challenges to diagnosis unless appropriate consideration is given to the impact of their sensory problems on cognitive development.

Sensory impairments commencing later in life resemble those that occur in the general population. Individuals with particular syndromes may be at special risk. For example, persons with Down syndrome are predisposed to hearing loss associated with aging, and to both cataracts and degenerative corneal changes as a result of keratoconus. Vision screening is now recommended for all adults with developmental disabilities every 5 years beyond the age of 45. Adults with mild or moderate intellectual impairments should have regular otoscopy and removal of earwax followed by audiometry or testing with whispered speech; those with severe intellectual disability should be screened utilizing otoacoustic emissions.

Mental health clinicians should be aware of psychopathology that is more common in persons with severe sensory impairments. Individuals who are blind (i.e., no more than light perception in both eyes and wearing glasses makes no difference) can present behaviourally with adjustment difficulties and are predisposed to both autism and problems with their sleep/wake cycle. Individuals who are deaf (i.e., hearing loss is sufficiently severe that they cannot process speech sounds auditorially) often experience tinnitus that needs to be distinguished from hallucinations. Sometimes the clinician will need advice from an informant aware of the "deaf culture" to distinguish the person's normal language structure from formal thought disorder. And deterioration in communication and sign fluency may be observed in those with sensory impairments who develop a psychotic disorder.

Clinicians should inform families about other services that can assist them. Both the Canadian National Institute for the Blind and the Canadian Hearing Society provide information and advisory services for families and individuals. Given the frequency of genetic disorders causing early onset hearing and visual impairment, clinicians should also refer families to professional genetic counselling services.

Further Readings:

Freeman, R. D., & Groenveld, M. (2000). The behaviour of children and youth with visual and hearing disability. In C. Gillberg & G. O'Brien (Eds.), *Developmental disability and behaviour* (pp. 27-47). London: Mac Keith Press.

Nagtzaam, L., & Vink, M. (1998). Visual and hearing impairment in people with intellectual disability. *Current Opinion in Psychiatry, 11*(5), 527-530.

1.4.3 Epilepsy

Epilepsy is a tendency to have recurrent seizures unprovoked by any immediately identifiable cause. A diagnosis of seizures is made on the basis of a careful description of the behavioural events and relevant investigations. Isolated seizures or a transient epileptic disorder may be seen in the presence of electrolyte or metabolic imbalances, drug withdrawal, infection of the nervous system, or sleep deprivation. And epilepsy needs to be distinguished from syncope, transient ischemic attacks, muscle spasms, narcolepsy, and movement disorders (e.g., tics, dystonia, and choreoathetosis). Psychogenic non-epileptic seizures should be considered in those with a history of physical or sexual abuse and borderline personality characteristics.

The rate of epilepsy in persons with intellectual disabilities is 25%, or 30 times the rate in the general population. It is especially high in those with cerebral palsy (50%) and in certain individual syndromes like tuberous sclerosis (90%). Onset of epilepsy in the first year of life is strongly linked to developmental delay. Infantile spasms in the neonatal period (West syndrome) can evolve into the Lennox-Gastaut syndrome (developmental disability and a mixture of seizure patterns including atypical absence, myoclonic jerks, atonic and tonic clonic). Up to one in four individuals with autism spectrum disorder develop seizures for the first time in late adolescence, and persons with Down syndrome frequently develop seizures for the first time in concert with Alzheimer's dementia in their 50s.

Recent studies are beginning to shed light on the relationship between epilepsy and dual diagnosis. Neuroses and affective disorders occur in 28% of those with intellectual disability and epilepsy, a rate twice that seen in persons with intellectual disability alone. Psychoses, often paranoid in nature, occur in 10% of individuals with intellectual disability and epilepsy. Dual diagnosis is more frequent in those with greater seizure severity and frequency, and in those at lower risk to lose consciousness during seizures. Somewhat surprisingly, problem behaviours are found to be less frequent in those with seizures. When behaviour problems do occur, clinicians should explore the possibility that these are caused by anticonvulsant medications, particularly phenobarb, primidone, or diphenlhydantion.

Poorly controlled epilepsy is a significant factor in increased caregiver burden and reduced quality of life for the individual with developmental disability. Although contemporary practice aims for anticonvulsant monotherapy in 85% of the general population, this is achieved in only 60% of the population with intellectual disabilities. The importance of regular meals and adequate sleep with prompt treatment of intercurrent illness or constipation should not be minimized. When psychotropic medications are indicated, those like phenothiazines and tricyclinc antidepressants, known to reduce the seizure threshold, ought to be avoided. The contribution of psychotherapy in individual cases should also be considered—embarrassment about seizures, fear of injury or death, and social isolation are frequently encountered themes in those with mild or moderate intellectual impairment. Information and peer support from epilepsy associations can be helpful to individuals and caregivers alike.

Further Readings:

Coulter, D. L. (1997). Comprehensive management of epilepsy in persons with mental retardation. *Epilepsia, 38*(Suppl. 4), S24-S31.

Espie, C. A. S., Watkins, J., Curtice, L., Espie, A., Duncan, R., Ryan, J. A., Brodie, M. J., Mantalka, & Sterrick, M. (2003). Psychopathology in people with epilepsy and intellectual disabilities: An investigation of potential explanatory variables. *Journal of Neurology, Neurosurgery, and Psychiatry, 74*(11), 1485-1492.

Reuber, M., & Elger, C. E. (2003). Psychogenic nonepileptic seizures: Review and update. *Epilepsy and Behaviour, 4*(3), 205-216.

1.4.4 Cerebral Palsy

Cerebral palsy includes a range of non-progressive syndromes of posture and motor impairment that result from an insult to the developing central nervous system. Although obstetric factors and perinatal anoxia were first thought to cause cerebral palsy, in 1897 Sigmund Freud (a child and adult neurologist before turning to psychoanalysis) drew attention to problems with early brain development, an approach that is the basis of present-day classifications.

Children who develop cerebral palsy are hypotonic in infancy, and the ultimate pattern of disability evolves over the next year or two. Fifty percent of cases involve spasticity, 20% athetosis, and the balance are "mixed" (including ataxia and rigidity). Intellectual disability occurs in 30–60% of individuals with cerebral palsy and is often severe in those individuals with spastic quadriplegia and seizures. The stress experienced by parents of children with cerebral palsy resembles that faced by parents of children with major congenital anomalies. Their children need physiotherapy, splinting, and various surgical procedures to optimize motor function. Child developmental clinics offer the supports and services of a multidisciplinary team of surgeons and therapists. Family support and guidance are important in preventing dependency and passivity in the younger child and reducing risks of potential stigmatization or discrimination in later years.

Attention problems and depression are often encountered in individuals with cerebral palsy. Mental health clinicians need to be aware of the risk of misidentifying depression as an "adjustment disorder." Psychotic disorders may occur but there is no published evidence of a predisposition; when psychotic symptoms do occur, they are treated in the traditional manner. Psychotherapy needs to include exploration of the individual's feelings about the disability, ways to enhance self-image and self-esteem, and guidance about how to appreciate the effect of one's behaviour on others and setting realistic and achievable goals for the future. Progress may be slow if the individual with a disability is using a communication board or other augmentative assistive devices, but the time spent can be highly beneficial both for the individual and for family and caregivers. Guidance for agency caregivers, who are more likely accustomed to caring for individuals with severe intellectual and physical impairments, is often needed when they find themselves dealing with an individual with mild intellectual impairment and severe mobility problems.

Clinicians also need to be vigilant for referrals that involve behaviour difficulties including anger, aggression, or self-injury because the individual with developmental disability may be experiencing unrecognized physical discomfort. Gastroesophageal reflux, muscle spasm, and uncomfortable seating (i.e., wheelchair positioning) are among a variety of the causes of behavioural changes. Once these concerns are appropriately managed, the behaviour difficulties will likely subside.

FURTHER READINGS:

Harris, J. C. (1995). *Developmental neuropsychiatry: Assessment, diagnosis and treatment of developmental disorders* (Vol. 2). New York: Oxford University Press.

Koman, L. A., Paterson Smith, B., & Shilt, J. S. (2004). Cerebral palsy. *Lancet, 363*, 1619-1631.

1.5 To understand the comorbid mental health problems that influence the adjustment and quality of life of persons with developmental disabilities

At least 40% of individuals with an intellectual disability have an additional mental disorder, a rate 3 or 4 times greater than observed in members of the general population. Some psychiatric illnesses, like schizophrenia, are more prevalent, and others, like substance abuse, are less prevalent than in the general population. Some disorders, for example, self-injury and pica, are rarely seen other than in persons with a severe intellectual disability. Like the medical comorbidities considered in Section 1.4, mental health comorbidities have an added impact on the individual's adaptive problems beyond that of their primary cognitive impairment. Accordingly, treatment and support aimed at eliminating or modifying the impact and severity of mental disorders must be included in a treatment-management plan designed to address adaptive problems and enhance quality of life.

In what follows, DC-LD, an innovative approach to the diagnosis and categorization of mental disorders developed by the UK Royal College of Psychiatrists, provides a conceptual base and framework. The manual identifies five categories or "levels" of psychiatric disorder. While detailed consideration of the full range of mental disorders occurring in persons with developmental disabilities is beyond the scope of this guide, the following subsections outline the major categories of comorbidity.

Further Reading:

Royal College of Psychiatrists. (2001). *DC-LD: Diagnostic criteria for psychiatric disorders for use with adults with learning disabilities/mental retardation.* London: Gaskell.

1.5.1 Diagnostic and Nosologic Challenges

Clinicians familiar with mental disorders in the general population need to modify their approaches to the diagnosis and categorization of these disorders in individuals with intellectual disabilities. Intellectual and communication impairments predispose these individuals to atypical presentations. These presentations reflect the pathoplastic effects of the intellectual impairment on the signs and symptoms of the mental disorders. Indeed, in those with severe intellectual impairment and major communication problems, such presentations can be essentially "behavioural" in nature. In these circumstances, common mental disorders like anxiety and depression may be misdiagnosed as "challenging behaviours." In order to minimize this risk and to ensure a systematic approach to assessment, DC-LD employs a step-wise procedure:

1. Identify the level of intellectual impairment (recorded on Axis I).
2. Identify the causes of the intellectual impairment, where possible (recorded on Axis II).
3. Identify the level of psychiatric disorder utilizing diagnostic categories listed in the DC-LD manual (recorded on Axis III).

Sections 1.1 and 1.2 have provided the relevant background for Axis I and II. Subsections 1.5.2–1.5.6 now provide background for identifying the five levels of psychiatric disorder recorded on Axis III of the DC-LD manual. Appendix B provides a format for recording the assessments.

Those clinicians interested in similar DSM-IV diagnostic categories should note that the DC-LD manual has appropriate cross-referencing procedures. And those not considering the use of DC-LD will be interested to know that the USA National Association for the Dually Diagnosed (NADD) has published a manual, DM-ID (see the reading below), directed at modifying DSM-IV categories for use with individuals with intellectual disabilities.

FURTHER READING:

Fletcher, E., Loschen, E., Stavrakaki, C., & First, M. (Eds.). (2007). *Diagnostic manual – intellectual disability: A clinical guide for diagnosis of mental disorders in persons with intellectual disability.* New York: NADD Kingston.

Wing, L., & Gould, J. (1979). Severe impairments of social interaction and associated abnormalities in children: Epidemiology and classification. *Journal of Autism and Developmental Disorders*, *9*(1), 11-29.

1.5.2 Level A: Pervasive Developmental Disorders

In 1979 Wing and Gould proposed to accommodate a group of specific syndromes, including those first delineated by Leo Kanner (1943) and Hans Asperger (1944), under the "autism spectrum disorder" concept. Autism spectrum disorders are characterized by a triad of impairments of social interaction, communication, and imagination associated with a narrow, repetitive range of activities. This triad of social impairments can be seen in individuals at any level of intellectual functioning. Profiles of abilities are typically patchy, occasionally showing one remarkable isolated skill in those referred to as "autistic savants."

A diagnosis of pervasive developmental disorders (PDD) was introduced in 1980 in DSM-III and subsequently used as well in the *International Classification of Diseases* (ICD-10) and DC-LD as an alternative to autism spectrum disorder. Fragile X syndrome and tuberous sclerosis are two well-established genetic disorders that involve a significant risk for autistic features.

These disorders seem to be increasing in prevalence, and there is concern that the increase could be associated with the use of thimerosal-containing vaccines. However, a Montreal study (Lazoff, Zhong, Piperni, & Fombonne, 2010) has concluded that the discontinuation of thimerosal use in vaccines in 1996 has not influenced the risk of these disorders. Research continues, particularly in genetics, to establish etiological factors. The Montreal study observed a prevalence of 79.1 per 10,000 school children, composed of 25.4 for autistic disorder, 43.6 for PDD-NOS (not otherwise specified), 9.7 for Asperger syndrome, and 0.4 for childhood disintegrative disorder.

The various pervasive developmental disorders are identified and described first in children. In adults, the unique behavioural features seen in childhood persist but may be less obvious to mental health professionals. If a careful developmental history is not recorded in adults, diagnostic errors are likely.

In general, the earlier the onset and greater the severity of symptoms, the greater the likelihood of life-long disability. Accordingly, in what follows, those with an early onset and a poor prognosis for independence (i.e., childhood disintegrative disorder, Rett syndrome, and most cases of Kanner's "autistic" syndrome) are considered together, leaving the others (Asperger syndrome and "high-functioning" autism) in a separate grouping.

Childhood Disintegrative Disorder

Childhood disintegrative disorder is extremely rare (1 per 100,000). Males are more susceptible than females (3:1). There is a period of normal development from birth to 30 months, then a period of severe behavioural regression lasting 1–3 years, leaving an individual with severe or profound developmental disability but relatively good motor skills.

Rett Syndrome

Rett syndrome is more common (1 per 15,000). It affects females almost exclusively, but has a similar natural history. There is a rapid developmental regression between 1 and 4 years of age with loss of purposeful movement, characteristic "hand-wringing" movements, episodes of hyperventilation, seizures, and preserved eye contact. Ambulation is usually lost, and the clinician will encounter adults who require wheelchair assistance and who may also be somewhat spastic and scoliotic. Rett syndrome, linked to a mutation of the MECP2 gene on Xq28, is coded on Axis II of DC-LD and described in Appendix I of the DC-LD manual in a list of "behavioural phenotypes."

Kanner's Autistic Syndrome

Autism, which is more common in males, may be suspected because of poor attachment and social interactions in infancy; it is usually not diagnosed until 18–30 months. Kanner's original criteria—failure to interact, "tendency to preserve sameness," and delayed/absent development of language—are reflected in the content of screening instruments (e.g., Checklist for Autism in Toddlers) and observation assessment scales (e.g., Autism Diagnostic Observation Schedule). Early diagnosis facilitates early behavioural strategies (e.g., intensive behavioural intervention) that may reverse some of the child's inability to socially interact and facilitate learning in the preschool years. If such improvement is sustained, the numbers of individuals who may adapt successfully in adulthood (around 20%) may increase, but the research evidence on long-term prognosis is still limited. Meanwhile, the development of socially useful language by age 5 and higher intellectual functioning are the favoured prognostic indicators. Approximately 25% develop seizures in late adolescence/early adulthood.

Treatment methods. Psychiatrists and psychologists may be asked to consider pharmacotherapy treatment or behavioural interventions for those who appear anxious, suffer from "rage attacks," or have prominent obsessive-compulsive features. Pharmacologic treatment is "symptomatic" and should be undertaken on a case by case basis. High doses of vitamin B_6 (co-administered with magnesium and other B vitamins) may be helpful in selected cases, and naltrexone should be considered in those with severe self-injurious behaviour. Families of individuals with childhood disintegrative disorder, Rett syndrome, and autism require psychoeducation, social support, and often genetic advice. Future biomedical research will no doubt yield insights that will help to determine the risks of recurrence in families and, hopefully, will lead to interventions that are more than "symptomatic."

Asperger Syndrome and High-Functioning Autism

There is a continuing debate about how to distinguish high-functioning autism and Asperger syndrome, perhaps not surprising since both are included in the "autism spectrum" and sometimes individuals receive both diagnoses at different times in their lives. What is clear is the contrasting clinical picture of these disorders with the three disorders considered above. Diagnosis usually occurs later in childhood (e.g., age 11 years, 4 months, in a study of 100 males with Asperger syndrome reported by Cederlund and Gillberg, 2004). In adults who have not been diagnosed earlier, a variety of psychiatric diagnoses are reported including personality disorder, schizophreniform, or unspecified psychosis or affective disorder. Treatment with antipsychotics or other medications provides little benefit and can sometimes cause serious side effects. Clinical features like avoidance or poor quality eye contact, a monotone voice, odd or inappropriate affect, limited use of gesture, and insistence on "lecturing" about a favourite topic should alert the clinician to consider Asperger syndrome. Some individuals during adulthood are seen as "aloof" (with trouble tolerating the company of others), some seen as "active and odd" (talk and act strangely in social settings), and a few seen as "passive" (often passive-aggressive).

Treatment methods. Regardless of the pattern, individuals with Asperger syndrome and high-functioning autism are frequently misunderstood, and psychoeducation may be the clinician's most important contribution after making the diagnosis. In late adolescence or early adulthood, they may become significantly depressed as they begin to appreciate how different they are from peers. Supportive psychotherapy and sometimes antidepressant medications are beneficial at this stage. Novel antipsychotics at low doses may also be used if irritability and aggression are encountered. Lithium carbonate or anticonvulsant "mood stabilizers" are used in the treatment of those with co-existent mood disorders.

Individuals with motor-coordination problems should be referred for consultation to a physiotherapist. Individuals with sensory problems or difficulties in daily living skills should be referred to an occupational therapist. Speech and language therapists can help with communication problems and provide advice about how to deal with complex language encounters. Psychologists can explain abstract social rules to help individuals navigate stressful social situations. Structure, order, and routine are important and need to be encouraged in all interactions; abstractions and symbolism should be avoided.

Further Readings:

Berney, T. (2007). Mental health needs of children versus adults with autism spectrum disorders. *Advances in Mental Health and Learning Disabilities, 1*(4), 10-14.

Cederlund, M., & Gillberg, C. (2004). One hundred males with Asperger syndrome: A clinical study of background and associated factors. *Developmental Medicine and Child Neurology, 46*(10), 652-660.

Lazoff, T., Zhong, L., Piperni, T., & Fombonne, E. (2010). Prevalence of pervasive developmental disorders among children at the English Montreal School Board. *Canada Journal of Psychiatry, 55*(11), 715-720.

Tantam, D. (2003). The challenge of adolescents and adults with Asperger syndrome. *Child Adolescent Psychiatric Clinics of North America,* 12(1), 143-163.

Xenitidis, K., Pliokosta, E., Maltezos, S., & Papps, V. (2007). Assessment of mental health problems in people with autism. *Advances in Mental Health and Learning Disabilities, 1*(4), 15-22.

1.5.3 Level B: Psychiatric Illnesses

The particular psychiatric illnesses selected for consideration in this subsection are common and often responsive to therapeutic interventions once diagnosed accurately. Accordingly, emphasis is given to atypical presentations that can prevent accurate diagnosis and, therefore, preclude treatments that should be provided. In each instance, reference is made to relevant behavioural phenotypes.

Schizophrenia

The prevalence of schizophrenia in persons with intellectual disabilities is 3%, versus 1% in the general population. This increased risk may reflect a decline in intellectual function in people with schizophrenia—recall Kraepelin's term "dementia praecox"—or a neurodevelopmental predisposition to intellectual impairment (for which a 22q11 deletion, i.e., velocardiofacial syndrome, represents a "model" disorder), or both. In terms of symptomatology, DC-LD suggests that the diagnosis of schizophrenia is likely impossible in those with severe intellectual impairment and urges caution in characterizing delusions and hallucinations even in those with less severe cognitive impairment. For example, the content of delusions often reflects the developmental level and life experiences of these individuals (e.g., monsters, celebrities), and some "positive" symptoms (e.g., passivity phenomena, thought insertion) may be absent. An inclination to "self talk" should never be automatically equated with hallucinations since it can also be seen as part of certain behavioural phenotypes, for example Down syndrome. "Negative" symptoms like motivational problems, apathy, and indifference need to be differentiated from premorbid levels of adaptive behaviour.

Interventional studies of individuals with schizophrenia have observed longer intervals of hospital care, frequent use of combinations of conventional and atypical antipsychotic medications (including clozapine), and enhanced levels of community support following hospitalization. In such circumstances, psychoeducation and consistent levels of caregiver support will be important elements in treatment-management plans.

Mood Disorders

A 2004 UK study reported a sixfold increase in the risk for "chronic depressed mood" in adults who had been identified early in life as mildly intellectually impaired (Collishaw, Maughan, & Pickles, 2004). The authors listed socioeconomic disadvantage and ill health as important variables in explaining this risk. This study illustrates growing awareness that mood disorders are an important consideration in the lives of individuals with developmental disabilities. Assessment of each individual must involve careful review of the family history, the developmental and health histories as well as current stressors. For example, studies on bereavement show that this experience is often neglected in evaluating behavioural and mood changes. That behavioural changes are significant in mood disorders follows the important insights pioneered by Sovner and Hurley commencing in 1982.

In addition to the obvious or so-called vegetative symptoms (e.g., changes in appetite, sleep), clinicians need to be aware that an onset or increase in self-injury, a loss of ability in daily living skills, and irritability may be present in depression, and distractibility, non-compliance, and aggression in mania. Individuals with Down syndrome are somewhat predisposed to depression. Suicide is less common in individuals with developmental disabilities although a Canadian study reported that one third of adults with mental retardation reported suicidal ideation or thoughts "that life is not worth living." The full range of biomedical and psychosocial treatments available to treat mood disorders are employed in the care of persons with developmental disabilities; more common therapies include cognitive and dialectical behaviour therapy modified for the individual's level of intellectual functioning.

DC-LD Level B lists depressive episodes, manic episodes, and mixed affective episodes; if problem behaviours are prominent, they can be listed in Level D ("problem behaviours due to psychiatric illness").

Anxiety Disorders

The various anxiety disorders occurring in the general population are also common in individuals with intellectual disabilities. The DC-LD manual outlines clinical approaches to ensure that these disorders are recognized in practice. Because many individuals are unable to describe the subjective features involved, clinicians must rely on observable physiological features of anxiety like appearing frightened, sweating, trembling, and becoming flushed. Irritability, self-injury, or property destruction may also indicate an anxiety disorder, particularly in those unable to describe their worries or fears. Compulsions need to be distinguished from autistic behavioural traits or from rhythmic movements seen frequently in people with severe and profound intellectual impairment (i.e., stereotypies).

Anxiety associated with other psychiatric disorders (e.g., depression) or medical problems (e.g., hyperthyroidism) is usually classified separately from the main anxiety disorder subtypes like panic or agoraphobia.

Among the genetic disorders, the behavioural phenotype associated with Williams syndrome includes anxiety symptoms, some based on an inclination to overempathize with the feelings of others and a distinct hypersensitivity to sound. In a comprehensive review of anxiety problems, Bailey and Andrews (2003) reported that the fears of adults with intellectual disabilities are similar to those occurring in children of equivalent developmental age (e.g., fears of the supernatural or of animals). Once again, the interventions for anxiety disorders utilized in the general population can be applied in treating individuals with intellectual disabilities (e.g., CBT, SSRIs).

Attention Deficit Disorder

Within the category "hyperkinetic disorder," DC-LD lists two subtypes of attention-deficit hyperactivity disorder (ADHD): childhood onset and age of onset unknown. The DC-LD manual suggests that ADHD be diagnosed in adults when poor attention, impulsive and disorganized behaviour, and problems maintaining purposeful behaviour at levels beyond those expected in individuals with developmental disabilities are observed. Attentional problems are more prevalent in individuals with severe intellectual impairment. Psychostimulants and other medications used in mainstream practice are often prescribed.

Dementia

While dementia can occur in any individual with an intellectual disability, there is a clear and well-defined predisposition in those with Down syndrome; depressive symptoms and seizures are common comorbidities. Hypothyroidism, to which individuals with Down syndrome are also predisposed, is an important differential diagnosis. Combined medical and psychiatric follow-up are obviously necessary not only for the individual but also for caregivers, in offering guidance and support as the dementia progresses.

Post-Traumatic Stress Disorder

In a recent systematic review of the effects of various traumatizing life events on people with intellectual disabilities, Wigham, Halton, and Taylor (2011) note that the usual criteria for post-traumatic stress disorder need to be supplemented for those individuals to include behavioural problems, physical health changes, and changes in skill levels. For individuals who have experienced sexual abuse, behaviours such as inappropriate sexual remarks, withdrawal into fantasy, and sexual "acting out" may be observed. An important goal of treatment-management programs for traumatized individuals is to ensure not only that the trauma is not repeated but that it is acknowledged and validated for the victim irrespective of possible legal consequences.

Further Readings:

Bailey, N. M, & Andrews, T. M. (2003). Diagnostic criteria for psychiatric disorders for use with adults with learning disabilities/mental retardation (DC-LD) and the diagnosis of anxiety disorders: A review. *Journal of Intellectual Disabilities Research, 47* (Suppl.), 50-61.

Bouras, N., Marlin, G., Leese, M., Vanstralen, M., Holt, G., Thomas, C., ... Boardman, J. (2004). Schizophrenia-spectrum psychoses in people with and without intellectual disability. *Journal of Intellectual Disability Research, 48*(6), 548-555.

Collishaw, S., Maughan, B., & Pickles, A. (2004). Affective problems in adults with mild learning disability: the roles of social disadvantage and ill-health. *British Journal of Psychiatry, 185*, 350-351.

Gothelf, D., (2007). Velocardiofacial syndrome. *Child & Adolescent Psychiatric Clinics of North America, 16*, 677-693.

Lunsky,Y. (2004). Suidicidality in a clinical community sample of adults with mental retardation. *Research in Developmental Disabilities, 25*(3), 231-243.

Wigham, S., Halton, L., & Taylor, J. (2011). The effects of traumatizing life events in people with intellectual disabilities: A systematic review. *Journal of Mental Research in Intellectual Disabilities, 4*, 19-39.

1.5.4 Level C: Personality Disorders

Epidemiological Considerations

Surveys to establish the prevalence of personality disorders in persons with intellectual disabilities have encountered the predictable methodologic challenges (e.g., problems with definition, "self-report" difficulties, selective factors in clinical populations). Accordingly, widely discrepant frequency patterns have been observed. In spite of these challenges, experienced clinicians are well aware that personality disorders are frequent among referrals from families, agencies and, in particular, forensic services.

Categorization

The DC-LD manual recommends extreme care in diagnosing personality disorders. It suggests that the diagnosis not be made before age 21 to allow for lags in personality development and not ever in those with severe or profound intellectual impairment since diagnostic criteria cannot be fairly applied. In the first instance, the DC-LD manual sets out criteria for an "unspecified personality disorder" including the presence of traits that are chronic, pervasive, and maladaptive. It suggests that diagnosis of certain personality disorder subtypes (e.g., schizoid, avoidant, dependent) should be avoided in view of the difficulty in differentiating them from the intellectual disability. However, the manual lists other subtypes (e.g., paranoid, histrionic, and anakastic) that are more easily delineated.

Although any personality disorder may need to be accommodated in an individual's treatment-management plan, this is especially true for those with the dissocial and emotionally unstable borderline subtypes. The dissocial category is similar to the antisocial category found in the DM-ID, and includes

- callous unconcern for the feelings of others;
- gross and persistent irresponsibility and disregard for social norms, rules, and obligations;
- a low tolerance for frustration and low threshold for discharge of aggression, including violence; and
- incapacity to experience guilt or to profit from adverse experience.

In 1988, Hurley and Sovner published a review of borderline personality disorder in individuals with developmental disabilities. They described clinical features very similar to those seen in individuals without disabilities, recommended treatment strategies used in mainstream practice, and noted a pattern of spontaneous improvement and maturation in those in their 30s and 40s.

Clinicians should be aware of other diagnostic possibilities especially in individuals presenting with prominent aggressive and destructive propensities.

DC-LD Level D, concerned with "problem behaviours," includes a category where such behaviours can be listed as "due to a personality disorder." Sometimes behaviour problems such as "rage attacks" can be accommodated as part of a "behavioural phenotype" on Axis II (e.g., Fragile X syndrome). DM-ID provides suggestions about using the antisocial personality disorder category or "intermittent explosive disorder" within a broader category of "Impulse Control Disorders not elsewhere classified."

Treatment Methods

Various counselling or drug treatment approaches can be included in treatment-management plans for individuals, and psychoeducation for caregivers about personality disorders is important in every case where the diagnosis is made. Finally, readers will be interested in Simon Baron-Cohen's recent work wherein he expands his exposition of empathy problems observed in individuals with Asperger syndrome to individuals with borderline, narcissistic, and antisocial personality disorders. In particular, his suggestions about teaching empathy to younger people, thereby (one hopes) preventing later personality problems, are relevant to people with developmental disabilities.

FURTHER READINGS:

Alexander, R. T., Tajuddin, M., & Gangadharan, S. K. (2007). Personality disorders in intellectual disability: Approaches to pharmacotherapy. *Mental Health Aspects of Developmental Disabilities, 10*(4), 129-136.

Baron-Cohen, S. (2011). *The science of evil: On empathy and the origins of cruelty.* New York: Basic Books.

Coccaro, E. F., & McLoskey, M. S. (2010). Intermittent explosive disorder: Clinical aspects. In E. Aboujaoude & L. M. Koran (Eds), *Impulse control disorders* (pp. 221-232). Cambridge: Cambridge University Press.

Hurley, A. D., & Sovner, R. (1988). The clinical characteristics and management of borderline personality disorder in mentally retarded persons. *Psychiatric Aspects of Mental Retardation Reviews, 7*, 42-49.

Khan, A., Cowan, C., & Roy, A. (1997). Personality disorders in people with learning disabilities: A community survey. *Journal of Intellectual Disability Research, 41*(4), 324-330.

1.5.5 Level D: Problem Behaviours

Evolving Perspectives

Level D includes problem behaviours like aggression, self-injury, and destructiveness, which can be primary and therefore coded here, or associated with other medical and/or psychiatric disorders as outlined in the preceding subsections. This hierarchical approach to categorization in DC-LD aims to minimize the risk, mentioned previously, of misdiagnosing "behavioural presentations" as behaviour problems instead of recognizing these behaviours as characteristics of other disorders.

Sometimes problem behaviours are mild and of brief duration, perhaps in response to known one-time stressors. In these instances such behaviours might be referred to as "adjustment disorders" and coded in Level B. Sometimes Level D behaviours are recorded in offenders, most often in those who have committed infrequent "high impact" offenses. There is a separate category, "sexually inappropriate behaviour," for obscene communications, genital exposure, and even sexual assault that "results from under development of social skills, lack of sexual education, misinterpretation of a relationship and sexual frustration." Conflict with the law in persons with intellectual disabilities is also considered in Section 3.5.

Traditionally, problem behaviours in individuals with intellectual disabilities have been treated behaviourally or with antipsychotic medications. More recently, however, it has been recognized that a comprehensive interprofessional perspective is needed for success. As outlined by Tassé in 2006, functional behavioural assessments are now incorporated in a multimethod approach, including the following:

- personal/social history (e.g., recording of recent stresses),
- physical examination and medical history,
- evaluation of current medications and possible side effects or interaction effects,
- psychiatric evaluation, and
- functional behavioural assessment.

Weiss and Lunsky (2010) have observed that behavioural crises, often prompting referrals to hospital emergency rooms, occur when there is a serious disparity between the needs of the person with an intellectual disability and the provision of treatment and support in the service system to meet these needs.

Treatment and support directed at minimizing the impact of environmental stressors and of health and mental health disorders should be complemented by additional efforts to enhance the individual's "resilience," a factor often compromised but unfortunately also ignored in persons with intellectual disabilities. Among the factors involved in resilience are optimal nutrition, fitness, supportive interpersonal relationships, and spiritual beliefs. This broadened perspective on problem behaviours reminds healthcare providers and caregivers that success needs to include interventions to reduce stressors, treat illnesses, and enhance resilience. In subsection 2.1.3, an approach to formulating treatment-management plans that accommodates this broader perspective is considered.

The Glasgow Studies

Cooper and her colleagues have completed two studies in Glasgow, one on aggression and the other on self-injurious behaviour, that provide important insights about prevalence, natural history, and pathogenetic factors. Aggression—including physically aggressive behaviour, verbally aggressive behaviour, and destructive behaviour as defined in DC-LD—had a point prevalence of 9.8% and a 2-year remission rate of 27.7%. These behaviours were independently associated with lower ability, female gender, ADHD, and urinary incontinence. The point prevalence of self-injury was 4.9% with a 2-year remission rate of 38.2%. Self-injury was independently associated with lower ability and having ADHD or visual impairment. Down syndrome was underrepresented in both those with aggressive behaviour and those with self-injury.

FURTHER READINGS:

Cooper, S. A., Smiley, E., Allan, L. M., & Jackson, A. (2009). Adults with intellectual disabilities: Prevalence, incidence and remission of self-injurious behaviour, and related factors. *Journal of Intellectual Disability Research, 53*(3), 200-216.

Cooper, S. A., Smiley, E., Jackson, A., & Finleyson, J., Allan, L., Mantry, D., & Morrison, J. (2009). Adults with intellectual disabilities: Prevalence, incidence and remission of aggressive behaviour, and related factors. *Journal of Intellectual Disability Research, 53*(3), 217-232.

Tassé, M. (2006). Functional behavioural assessment in people with intellectual disabilities. *Current Opinion in Psychiatry, 19*, 475-480.

Weiss, J., & Lunsky, Y. (2010). Service utilization patterns in parents of youth and adults with intellectual disability who experienced behavioural crises. *Journal of Mental Health Research in Intellectual Disabilities, 3*, 145-163.

1.5.6 Level E: Other Disorders

DC-LD Level E describes psychiatric disorders that cannot be incorporated in Levels A–D. In this subsection, two categories are considered briefly to illustrate this option and to outline important clinical challenges.

Sleep Disorders

Sleep disorders are categorized in ICD-10 as "organic" (diseases of the nervous system) or "non-organic" (mental disorders). In persons with intellectual disorders, sleep disorders can occur at any age but tend to be most common in the early years of life. Sleep disorders appear more frequently in people with autism spectrum disorders, regardless of IQ levels. These individuals may have problems getting to sleep and staying asleep. In milder cases, strict appropriate bedtime routines (i.e., sleep hygiene) are recommended, while in more serious situations melatonin has been helpful. Obstructive sleep apnea is often encountered in individuals with Down syndrome and with Prader-Willi syndrome; a narcolepsy-like problem has also been observed in the latter. Coaching individuals with intellectual disabilities to utilize CPAP (continuous positive airway pressure) devices is a major challenge. Problems falling asleep, frequent and prolonged nocturnal awakenings, daytime somnolence, and bedwetting are frequent in persons with Smith-Magenis syndrome; either melatonin or acebutolol should be considered in these individuals.

Sexual Disorders

The DC-LD manual lists gender identity disorders, disorders of sexual preference, and psychological and behavioural disorders associated with sexual development and orientation in Level E, thereby offering several options for clinicians to use ICD-10 categories. Parkes and Hall (2006), in a comprehensive review of gender dysphoria and cross-dressing, recorded autism and aggression as significant comorbidities and suggested that clinicians "need to be open to considering gender dysphoria issues as a hidden etiology for presenting problems" (p. 268). They observe that cross-dressers with developmental disabilities are often isolated and stigmatized, indeed likely to experience suicidal rumination not unlike cross-dressers without disabilities.

Further Readings:

Parkes, G., & Hall, I. (2006). Gender dysphoria and cross-dressing in people with intellectual disability: A literature review. *Mental Retardation, 44*(4), 260-271.

Richdale, A. L. (1999). Sleep problems in autism, prevalence, cause and intervention. *Developmental Medicine & Child Neurology, 41*, 60-66.

Turk, J. (2003). Melatonin supplementation for severe and intractable sleep disturbance in young people with genetically determined developmental disabilities: Short review and commentary. *Journal of Medical Genetics, 40*(11), 793-796.

Part 2 – Skills

The skills outlined in the five sections that follow are best learned during an interval of supervised clinical practice, usually during post-graduate training. This interval should include experience in community, residential, and hospital settings thereby providing insights about the "continuum" of services needed by persons with developmental disabilities and dual diagnosis.

Skills and attitudes are best imparted together by instructors and mentors in university Academic Health Science Centres. These centres are linked with schools, developmental service agencies and social services, as well as with traditional hospital and community health agencies. Consequently, students experience the broad network of supports needed by children and adults with developmental disabilities over their lifetime. Indeed, learning about how to navigate and achieve optimal coordination of health services and social support is inherent in a high-quality curriculum.

Further Reading:

McKimm, J., & Brake, D. J. (2010). Interprofessional learning. *The British Journal of Hospital Medicine, 71*(10), 580-583.

2.1 To be familiar with how to prepare treatment-management plans for persons with developmental disabilities and dual diagnosis

This section reviews the special challenges involved in assessing individuals with developmental disabilities and in formulating treatment-management plans to address their complex needs.

"Treatment" and "management" are overlapping, yet distinct, facets of an intervention plan. Treatment is concerned with interventions that relate specifically to health and mental health problems that are diagnosed during clinical assessment. In contrast, management is linked conceptually to the developmental, case management, and social services needed by the individual with developmental disabilities and the caregivers as outlined in Section 1.3. Part of the synergy between treatment and management is the concept of resilience as briefly outlined in Section 1.5.4. Although resilience is often ignored in the design of treatment-management plans, those creating such plans should remain cognizant of the benefits of optimal nutrition, fitness, supportive interpersonal relationships, and spiritual beliefs in the lives of people with developmental disabilities. Interventions provided without comprehensive interprofessional assessments of need or without a thoughtful and carefully formulated treatment-management plan (renewed at least every 2 years) run the risk of reduced effectiveness, excessive cost, and potential harmfulness.

DC-LD serves as a user-friendly framework in bridging clinical diagnosis and formulating treatment-management plans for individuals with developmental disabilities (see Appendix B).

Clinical assessment is based on a bio-psycho-social model including the medical and developmental history described in Section 2.1.1 and on the physical and mental status examination, psychological evaluation, and rehabilitative assessments described in Section 2.1.2. The results of these assessments create a background and foundation for the formulation of effective interprofessional treatment-management plans.

2.1.1 Collecting the History

Although it is difficult to judge the relative importance of physical and mental status examinations, psychological and rehabilitative assessments, and special investigations in preparing treatment-management plans, there is little disagreement that the clinical history is the cornerstone of case formulation and diagnosis.

While some individuals with mild intellectual impairment can provide a basic history of their past and current life, they are usually regarded as "poor historians" because of impaired memory, comprehension problems, and difficulty communicating personal concerns. Accordingly, their contribution is often supplemented by information from other informants, like family members or agency staff. For persons with more severe intellectual and communication impairments, informants must provide all of the history. In both situations, copies of school, hospital, and social agency records are necessary to supplement information gathered directly.

In many clinics, a nurse or social worker is responsible for recording the "intake" history. Consents for release of records are necessary and should be obtained promptly from the individual or substitute decision maker. Sometimes a questionnaire is sent in advance to informants, but a personal interview is preferable to gather additional information about the daily life of the individual with developmental disability. A format for recording (i.e., not for collecting) a clinical history is provided in Appendix A. It can be used in instances where the primary focus of the assessment is "developmental" or where the primary focus is "dual diagnosis."

Once the basic "identifying information" has been recorded, the present concerns are reviewed. The family history may need to be expanded beyond the current generations if the individual is referred later to a genetics clinic.

As the interview proceeds, the interviewer will consider the need to obtain further healthcare records from other professionals and/or agencies.

Gathering and collecting a comprehensive and validated clinical history is time-consuming and labour intensive. Once the history is fully documented, it need only be updated when referrals occur or when there are significant changes in the individual's life. Such changes typically do occur in individuals with dual diagnosis, who experience cycles of deterioration and improvement over a period of years. As well, as noted in Section 1.3, the transitional periods from youth to adulthood and the adjustments that occur when the individual's parents or main caregivers die are important junctures for identifying "new" information.

The 2011 edition of *Tools for the Primary Care of People with Developmental Disabilities* includes formats for creating cumulative patient profiles, preventative care checklists, risk assessments in behavioural crises, and more.

Further Readings:

Levitas, A. S., & Silka, V. R. (2011). Mental health clinical assessment of persons with mental retardation and developmental disabilities: History. *Mental Health Aspects of Developmental Disabilities*, *4*(1), 31-42.

Medication Use Management Services. (2011). *Tools for the primary care of people with developmental disabilities*. Toronto: MUMs Guideline Clearing House. www.mumshealth.com

2.1.2 Conducting Clinical Examinations and Assessments

Completing a comprehensive clinical assessment of an individual with a developmental disability involves combining the history of the person and the direct observations of healthcare professionals. These professionals conduct clinical interviews along with more structured assessments particular to their disciplines.

Professionals need to understand how to modify their clinical interviews according to the individual's level of intellectual impairment and communication skills. Attention is given to these interview modifications in what follows.

At the outset of an interview with someone with mild intellectual impairment, healthcare professionals should inform and reassure the person about what is to occur during the clinical assessment. They should also explain consent and the limits of confidentiality (e.g., disclosing abuse). Thereafter, the question "Do you have any issues or problems that you think we should talk about?" is often a useful starting point, not only in reflecting the clinician's concern but in providing an opportunity to gauge the individual's insight and ability to communicate about such matters. The clinician must also be cognizant that most referrals are not self-initiated but reflect the perspective of a family member or caregiver.

As the interview proceeds, questions about feelings (e.g., sadness, anger, fear), and related anxiety and mood, can be introduced. Clinicians should use plain language and simplify the terminology. When prompting "yes/no" answers, the clinician should remember that those with developmental disabilities tend to acquiesce or respond affirmatively. It can be beneficial to use the individual's own words to explore emotions. To check later in the interview for reliability, the examiner can use comprehension checks or suggest the reverse of an earlier reply. Near the close of the interview, the clinician should ask for or provide the individual with a brief summary of the meeting, ask for the person's perspective on the discussion and whether there are any questions. The interview ends with an outline of what comes next for the individual, assuming he or she consents to further service.

When the individual is more severely intellectually impaired, the clinician establishes trust and rapport through "general conversation." During this social interaction, clinicians may make important observations. They obtain further details from caregivers.

The individual is usually seen with a family member or an agency support staff who can assist in reassuring the person, "interpreting" language or gestures that may be unfamiliar to the examiner, explaining the significance of unusual habits or mannerisms, and describing the "typical picture" of the individual. The examiner may use pictures or paper and pencil to invite the individual to identify numbers, sizes, shapes, and "social" situations. A series of booklets portraying common health issues and stressful situations like bereavement and abuse have been developed by Sheila Hollins, a UK psychiatrist with a special interest in communication and counselling for individuals with developmental disabilities. Even when verbal communication is quite limited or absent, facial expressions and body language can provide an important indication of awareness, attitudes, and positive or negative feelings attached to significant topics.

Individuals with features of autism spectrum disorders are often especially challenging for clinical interviewers. While they may appear disengaged or "aloof," many are really very anxious when being interviewed or examined by a stranger. They may respond with anything from apparent lack of interest, stereotypies, or perseverative questioning through to severe anger or aggression, putting themselves or others at risk. The clinician should rely on others who know the individual's characteristic responses and tolerance of questioning in judging how far to proceed in interviewing or prompting direct interactions.

Physicians or psychiatrists conduct physical and mental status examinations as part of their assessment. Any tradition that might suggest that a mental status examination be reserved only for individuals with dual diagnosis should be ignored in the case of those with significant intellectual and communication impairments. Given the prevalence of "behavioural presentations" like social withdrawal or irritability in individuals with common medical problems like GERD or constipation, clinicians need to be absolutely clear about the relevance of combining observations from the physical and mental status perspectives. A further overlap between mental health and physical observations is exemplified in the case of genetic syndromes with characteristic physical and behavioural features. For example, people with velocardiofacial syndrome may have significant physical problems (e.g., congenital heart anomalies) and mental health problems (e.g., schizophrenia); ignoring either in preparing a comprehensive treatment-management plan would be short-sighted for the individual's care.

Psychologists and rehabilitation therapists use standardized assessments as part of their evaluations. Although often not standardized on individuals with developmental disabilities, various psychological and rehabilitative assessments (e.g., intellectual and adaptive ability tests) are administered to supplement the clinical interview. Caution is needed in interpreting the results of these assessments and applicability to the normative group (i.e., expected developmental ability and chronological age). For psychological evaluation, more developmentally appropriate child assessments may be used due to their simple instructions and less reliance on verbal responses. For rehabilitation assessments, clinicians must take into account that individuals with developmental disabilities need to be evaluated for potential skill acquisition rather than skill loss and possible remediation.

Further Readings:

Al-Sheikh, A., & O'Hara, J. (2008). Psychiatric and mental status assessment in learning disabilities. *Advances in Mental Health and Learning Disabilities*, *2*(4), 21-28.

Dagnan, D. (2008). Psychological assessment for people with learning disabilities and mental ill-health. *Advances in Mental Health and Learning Disabilities*, *2*(4), 4-8.

Dwyer, J., & Reep, J. (2008). How occupational therapists assess adults with learning disabilities. *Advances in Mental Health and Learning Disabilities*, *2*(4), 9-14.

Levitas, A. S., DesNoyers Hurley, A., & Pary, R. (2001). The mental status examination in patients with mental retardation and developmental disabilities. *Mental Health Aspects of Developmental Disabilities*, *4*(1), 2-16.

2.1.3 Formulating Treatment-Management Plans

In recent decades, community-based healthcare has become a central aspect of social inclusion policy in the care of persons with developmental disabilities. Since the integration of these individuals in mainstream health, education, and social service agencies, the importance and necessity of treatment-management plans have become obvious to all involved. Coordination of effort on behalf of individuals with complex needs is neither automatic nor easily achieved within this "mainstream" service model. This subsection addresses the challenges entailed in creating a one-time, an intermittent, or an ongoing plan that will guide the efforts of caregivers and healthcare professionals.

Four essential steps in formulating a treatment-management plan are listed below:

- Summarize the individual's clinical difficulties from the perspective of the client and referrer.
- Outline the developmental, biomedical, and psychosocial factors that cause, or contribute significantly to, the individual's disabilities and therefore need to be addressed in preparing the treatment-management plan.
- List the developmental services and both the biomedical and psychosocial treatments relevant to optimal care for the individual.
- Analyze the prognostic considerations that relate to successful implementation of the treatment-management plan.

Creating a succinct summary of the individual's clinical problems, given the comprehensive assessments available from the clinical history and examination, is perhaps the most important step. The summary should include clinical items that are strategically important in identifying the pathogenetic factors that must be addressed in the interventions to follow. An omission is obviously a major problem.

An effective treatment-management plan will prioritize supports and treatment needed over the next 2 years (at the most), setting aside for later consideration items that can safely wait. Since clinical diagnosis is a key issue in formulation of treatment-management plans, normally professionals who are licensed to provide diagnoses (e.g., physicians, clinical psychologists) are given this responsibility. However, all members of an interdisciplinary team (Section 2.2) should be consulted and involved in the formulation of the plan.

Four categories of pathogenetic factors (biological, psychological, social, and developmental) are identified in DC-LD that should be part of the treatment-management plan. These factors are derived from research on the potential causes of individual disorders, and they provide a useful bridge and framework for listing interventions that will benefit the individual. This approach has already been discussed (Section 1.3) in identifying developmental, case management, and social service interventions linked to the individual's primary and secondary healthcare needs.

So how is resilience included in this approach? Although resilience issues have been researched for many years, it is only recently that serious attention has been given to including these important factors in the preparation of treatment-management plans. This "resilience" goal is addressed in a 2011 review by Herrman et al.:

> The most significant clinical application of the (resilience) concept is a reminder about the value of the clinician taking a good history and the need for developing a strong therapeutic alliance, the basic elements of a clinical encounter that can receive less attention in the professional era of biodeterminism, and emphasis on models and techniques in therapies. Based on knowledge of the factors that usually enhance resilience and how the patient has dealt with severe stress in the past, the clinician can reinforce optimal responses to adversity. (p. 263)

Accordingly, attention to nutrition, fitness, interpersonal relationships, and spiritual beliefs is necessary in the design of the treatment-management plan as the various developmental services and biomedical/psychosocial treatments are identified.

The rationale for including prognostic factors in a treatment-management plan is linked to the goal of achieving success in its implementation over the projected interval of delivery. Apart from factors associated directly with the individual with developmental disability (e.g., level of intellectual impairment, severity of health/mental health problems), several important external factors may influence the prognosis. These include the availability of needed resources (e.g., follow-up, funding, trained caregivers and professional staff), optimal interdisciplinary teamwork, ensuring compliance, and monitoring progress.

Often neglected in contemporary practice is the importance of advocacy, not only on behalf of individuals with developmental disabilities and their caregivers but also on a systemwide basis. Well-designed treatment-management plans must consider issues of advocacy whether in respect to a particular individual or more broadly to prevent professionals and agencies from different sectors operating in "silos."

Readers are referred to Appendix B, which sets out a framework for formulating treatment-management plans. It accommodates both the results of the comprehensive clinical assessment and the broad developmental and healthcare interventions needed by individuals with developmental disabilities and dual diagnosis.

Further Reading:

Herrman, H., Stewart, D., Diaz-Granados, & Berger, E., Jackson, B., & Yuen, T. (2011). In Review: What is resilience? *Canadian Journal of Psychiatry*, *56*(5), 258-265.

2.2 To be familiar with the necessity of interprofessional collaboration in providing care and support for persons with developmental disabilities and dual diagnosis

As outlined in Section 2.1.3, the skills of a number of professional disciplines are needed in assessing individuals with developmental disabilities and dual diagnosis who are referred to a clinic. Similarly, various professionals can be involved in implementing the treatment-management plan. This section discusses the interprofessional, collaborative teamwork that is needed to ensure that the plan is delivered appropriately. The discussion draws upon examples of interdisciplinary teamwork in London, United Kingdom; New Jersey, United States; and Ontario, Canada.

Two categories of teamwork are commonly practised:

Multidisciplinary – Members of two or more health disciplines, drawing on their own discipline's body of knowledge, work separately to achieve discipline-related clinical goals.

Interprofessional – Members of two or more health disciplines, using a systematic and integrated approach based on their respective health discipline's knowledge, work together to achieve common interprofessional clinical goals.

Because of the complex needs of people with developmental disabilities, interprofessional teamwork is the preferred approach. Obviously, teams may use overlapping approaches or evolve from one category to the other. Most healthcare professionals would agree that interprofessional teamwork requires specific education and attention to ensuring optimal collaboration between disciplines, and that such attention will ultimately benefit the "consumers" (i.e., the individuals and their caregivers) of the clinical service. Section 3.3 elaborates on interprofessional identities and attitudes that influence teamwork in the field of developmental disabilities.

Bouras and Holt (2010) trace the development of interprofessional clinical teams in Kent and southeast London following the closure of Darenth Park Institution, which served the area until 1981. Initially, Community Learning Disability Teams were created; each consisted of health and social service professionals expected to respond to a variety of complex problems, from social care to primary healthcare and tertiary mental healthcare. By 1983, it had become clear that individuals with dual diagnosis could not always be successfully integrated in mainstream mental health services. Accordingly, a specialized Mental Health in Learning Disabilities service was established that, along with a Challenging Behaviour team, continues to serve the region. It appears that the challenges of ensuring effective primary healthcare across the UK continue; an independent enquiry (Michael, 2008; see Section 1.4) has generated several recommendations, now being implemented, for better professional training, service delivery, and monitoring.

A somewhat similar model of care is practised in New Jersey (Criscione, Kastner, O'Brien, & Nathanson, 1994). A Developmental Disabilities Centre was first established at the Morristown Memorial Hospital in 1982. The centre's interprofessional team provides direct primary care as well as specialized medical care and consulting services to support primary care physicians and developmental service agencies across the state. The team includes collaborative mental healthcare in its mandate and ensures continuity of clinical care when an individual needs admission to hospital, dental care, and genetics assessments. Nurse practitioners have been assigned a central role in facilitating and coordinating the contributions of all team members to the individual's support plan.

Services in both London and New Jersey include training and research endeavours, along with clinical services, to ensure capacity building within the community.

In 2008, the Ontario government passed the Social Inclusion Act to promote care in the community for people with developmental disabilities. The act is primarily concerned with funding social supports, not healthcare. Although the act describes the necessity of services provided by psychologists, social workers, and speech-language pathologists (i.e., "specialized and professional services"), the legislation is silent on the need for interprofessional teamwork and collaborative healthcare services. Apart from five inpatient units for persons with dual diagnosis and limited outpatient consultation teams, there is little evidence that the Ministry of Health and Long-Term Care has made any specialized provisions for serving the long-term needs of adults with developmental disabilities.

For children and youth with dual diagnosis, healthcare teams in Ontario's Child Development Centres provide support. But beyond this age, families and agency caregivers are often left entirely without the kind of assistance available in the London and New Jersey models. Observations by Burge (2009) on Ontario's assertive community treatment teams and by Weiss and Lunsky (2010) on behavioural crises leave the distinct impression that there is serious neglect of adults with dual diagnosis in mainstream settings. As well, neither of the key ministries has addressed the current gaps in the training of healthcare professionals about developmental disabilities and the importance of interprofessional teamwork in correcting the current marginalization and neglect.

Further Readings:

Bouras, N., & Holt, G. (Eds.). (2010). *Mental health services for adults with intellectual disability: Strategies and solutions.* Hove, UK: Psychology Press.

Burge, P. (2009). Assertive community treatment teams and adults with intellectual disabilities. *Journal of Developmental Disabilities, 15*(3), 96-102.

Criscione, T., Kastner, T., O'Brien, D., & Nathanson, R. (1994). Replication of a managed health care initiative for people with mental retardation living in the community. *Mental Retardation, 32*(1), 43-52.

Morris, S. (2005). Specialized inpatient mental health units in Ontario. *Mental Health Aspects of Developmental Disabilities, 8*(3), 70-76.

Weiss, J., & Lunsky, Y. (2010). Service utilization patterns in parents of youth and adults with intellectual disability who experienced behavioural crisis. *Journal of Mental Health Research in Intellectual Disabilities, 3*, 145-163.

2.3 To be familiar with the provision of effective caregiver support in treatment-management plans for persons with developmental disabilities and dual diagnosis

The importance of an effective working relationship between healthcare professionals and the caregivers of persons with developmental disabilities cannot be overestimated. In this section, various facets of caregiver support including psychoeducation, guidance about treatments, and case-management liaison will be considered. Readers will also be interested in attitudinal variables that affect caregiver support as outlined in Section 3.3.

Although the majority of agency caregivers will have been educated about developmental disabilities during their training, the same cannot be said about family caregivers. The diagnosis of a developmental disability usually occurs in childhood and is rarely other than stressful for the parents and members of the extended family. Once the stress reactions have abated, there is a thirst for information that evolves as the individual with disabilities gets older.

Providing diagnostic information for family members is, in the first instance, a medical responsibility. Parents will ask how the diagnosis is made, what kind of confirmatory investigations are relevant, and for a prognosis of the child's expected developmental achievements. Ideally, both parents should be present when the clinician explains the diagnosis, given the impact on the family. The clinician should arrange a follow-up visit within a week or two to review information, confirm what details are understood, and deal with additional questions that inevitably arise in the interim. As part of the initial diagnosis, the clinician must explain to parents that the nature of the child's disability will change over time. The support plan will evolve and need revision in keeping with this developmental perspective.

In later years, parents will retain vivid memories of these initial medical interactions, both the positive and the unfortunate negative experiences. When they recall that the physician spent time with them, used simple non-technical language, and was empathetic, these memories are treasured. Well-informed parents will usually pass on relevant information to siblings, grandparents, and other family members, but if they report difficulties in conveying such information, the physician should assist. When a "syndrome" diagnosis is possible, the clinician can refer caregivers to the organization website (e.g., Down Syndrome Association) and share brochures and other publications.

Family physicians or pediatricians supporting and educating families with a child recently diagnosed with a developmental disability may enlist the assistance of other professionals. A psychologist or psychiatrist should be consulted when the parents exhibit poor child-rearing skills, psychiatric illness, alcohol problems, marital conflict, or other parental risk factors. If there is evidence of serious neglect of the child, a social worker from the Children's Aid Society should be called. In complex cases, a social worker usually assumes a case manager role to coordinate efforts to help the child and family. Resources and supports like a child disability allowance and regular respite with a foster family or group home need to be considered in every case.

A psychiatric disorder associated with an intellectual disability can occur at any age. Regardless of the age of onset, a dual diagnosis constitutes a source of burden beyond that linked to the developmental disability. Parents describe their adjustment to the dual diagnosis as a reiteration of what they faced when the intellectual disability was first diagnosed. Accordingly, mental health professionals can expect similar inquiries from parents such how the diagnosis is made, what the significant etiological factors are, and the potential prognosis. The parental needs for information about treatment and case management are intensified by a dual diagnosis.

As mentioned in Section 2.2, an interprofessional approach to care is desirable. Often available for children and youth, collaborative teams are less frequently available in Canada for adults, many of whom require continuing care to live with their parents. Transitional planning is necessary for young adults who are maturing physically and sexually, who are leaving school and ready for further education/work, and who may wish to live apart from their parents. Clinicians should refer individuals to "intensive" case management during this often stressful time.

Burdo-Hartman and Patel (2005) have published a useful account of a "medical home" model and transition planning for youth with disabilities. The medical home approach was first proposed in 1967 at the annual meeting of the American Academy of Pediatrics to provide "healthcare that is accessible, family oriented, continuous, comprehensive, coordinated, compassionate and culturally effective." In October 2009, the College of Family Physicians of Canada called on the federal government to adopt the model for all Canadians, not only those with disabilities and chronic illnesses.

Because agency caregivers are trained in developmental disabilities and sometimes dual diagnosis, psychoeducation is less important for them than for family caregivers. Yet agency staff still benefit from guidance about treatment and case management through liaison with healthcare professionals.

Broadhurst and Mansell (2007) found evidence for the importance of caregiver support in their study on factors contributing to the breakdown of residential placements for people with intellectual disabilities. They observed that a primary factor in placement breakdowns was not severe behaviour problems but lack of "external professional support" for caregivers, along with inadequate levels of training and managerial supervision. British psychologist Nancy Sheppard has documented the benefits of ongoing training and regular team meetings in providing for optimal care of individuals with a dual diagnosis. She describes three phases for "process consultations":

- raising awareness and developing understanding of the emotional needs of clients/service users,
- thinking about emotional reactions to clients, for example helping people to recognize transference and counter-transference feelings, and
- explaining group processes and helping staff to apply some of the group processes to their "group" (i.e., clients and staff).

FURTHER READINGS:

Broadhurst, S., & Mansell, J. (2007). Organizational and individual factors associated with breakdown of residential placements for people with intellectual disabilities. *Journal of Intellectual Disability Research, 51*, 4293-4301.

Burdo-Hartman, W., & Patel, D. (2005). Medical home and transition planning for children and their youth with special health care needs. *Pediatric Clinics of North America, 55*, 1287-1297.

Ryan, S. (1995a). Talking to the parents of a baby who is likely to develop permanent neurological impairment following a brain insult in the perinatal period. *Postgraduate Medical Journal, 71*, 336-340.

Ryan, S. (1995b). Telling the parents their child has severe congenital abnormalities. *Postgraduate Medical Journal, 71*, 529-537.

Sheppard, N. (2003). Working with care staff and organizations. In S. Hodges (Ed.), *Counselling adults with learning disabilities* (pp. 156-161). Basingstoke: Palgrave-MacMillan.

2.4 To be familiar with the provision of ambulatory treatment-management plans for people living in community residences

In this section, treatment-management for individuals who are living in a community residence is considered. The categorization of interventions already adopted in Section 2.1.3 and the framework illustrated in Appendix B are used to provide an outline for the review.

2.4.1 Developmental Services

Developmental services offer a range of supports for individuals, as determined by the person's level of intellectual impairment and adaptive abilities. Some individuals are mildly impaired, needing only minimal support, while others with profound difficulties need 24/7 "intensive" assistance.

In most jurisdictions in Canada (except Quebec), developmental services and healthcare services are administered by separate ministries. This is a meaningless distinction for persons with intellectual disabilities themselves but an important one for caregivers and healthcare professionals who need to cooperate and collaborate across two fields of endeavour. Indeed, for healthcare professionals, one of the important skills required for success—usually learned best through supervised clinical placements during their training—is how to relate to and support caregivers who provide for their clients and how to advocate for and navigate relevant services. Some of the attitudinal issues are considered in Section 3.2.

A Place to Live

A place to live involves accommodation, supervision, interpersonal relationships, and opportunities to develop and practise social and daily living skills. The developmental and social services sector is responsible for maintaining a range of residential options. Healthcare professionals will need to consider their client's residence as a potential contributor to health problems (from homelessness through optimal arrangements, to excessive supervision causing despair) and as a source of help in implementing treatment plans (from first aid to maintaining regular medication regimes). In addition, nutrition and exercise that support rehabilitation and foster resilience are often provided within an individual's residence.

Meaningful Activities

Meaningful activities is a phrase for referring to the range of education, training, work, and recreational pursuits that are tailored to the particular needs and aspirations of the individual with developmental disabilities. During the institutional era, efforts to "normalize" people's experience of the rhythms of life (e.g., over the 24-hour cycle, over the week, and over the seasons) often went astray. The policies of "community care" and social integration aim to avoid the depersonalization and routines of institutional living. From the perspective of healthcare professionals, once again vocational and leisure activities can be a source of difficulty or an avenue for treatment and improved resilience.

Perhaps the L'Arche communities best exemplify provision of supportive interpersonal relationships and spirituality. Unfortunately, healthcare professionals will regularly encounter examples of the chronic underfunding of support services for people with developmental disabilities. As a result, individuals may report depressed mood, boredom, and anxiety about their futures. In these circumstances, providing psychological support and systemic advocacy can be helpful.

Caregiver Support

As already suggested, learning to cooperate and liaise effectively with caregivers is a key professional skill for healthcare providers serving individuals with developmental disabilities. Caregivers are a critical source of "background support" in the individual's clinical history, and usually assist in implementing treatment recommendations and participate directly in health monitoring and intervention activities. Conversely, caregivers (even those trained in providing developmental services) are dependent on healthcare professionals for psychoeducation, guidance about treating health and mental health problems, and providing monitoring and prompt attention in the event of a health crisis.

Clinicians should refer family caregivers to providers of respite care. For families in particular, regular breaks from the usual responsibilities may be essential for physical and mental health.

Collaboration

Caregivers and healthcare professionals face important issues of time management. Caregivers have a myriad of daily support responsibilities beyond of the person's healthcare needs. Moreover, many individuals with developmental disabilities relate to their health professionals through caregivers, who may expect and need extra time. Accordingly, there needs to be appropriate attention to how and when caregivers and health professionals communicate, and both need to consider carefully how the individual is included and accommodated in discussions (in keeping with levels of capacity; see Section 3.5).

Not unlike the general population, visits to clinics and hospital often provoke anxiety in individuals with intellectual disabilities, and so clinicians should make every attempt to visit them in their own homes, or at least in familiar surroundings. In efforts to improve community and hospital care in the UK, user-friendly "hospital passports" (to convey important information about the individual) and nurse liaison specialists (in intellectual disability) have been introduced.

FURTHER READINGS:

Ferguson, D., & Scott, J. (2008). Spirituality, mental health and people with learning disabilities. *Advances in Mental Health and Learning Disabilities*, *2*(2), 37-41.

Vanier, J. (2007). *Our life together: A memoir in letters.* Toronto: Harper Perennial.

2.4.2 Psychosocial Treatments

The three categories of intervention discussed in this subsection are provided by therapists whose clinical skills relate to various aspects of adaptive behaviour and psychosocial functioning (e.g., communication, daily living skills, and interpersonal relationships). Although clinical diagnosis is important and relevant, facilitating improved levels of adaptation and optimal function is the primary focus of treatment. At intervals during treatment, adaptive and psychological functioning are reassessed to ensure progress or to revise the approach to be more effective. Although therapists may practice independently, in the field of developmental disabilities an interprofessional collaborative team approach is necessary and in the long-term more successful and sustainable for the individual and caregivers.

Behaviour Management

Behaviour management interventions have evolved significantly over the past 30–40 years. Initially called "behaviour modification" and limited to reinforcing desired behaviours and punishing undesired behaviours, this evolution of applied behaviour analysis has led to approaches based on "functional behavioural assessments." Functional behavioural assessments establish clear operational definitions of target behaviours, analyze the behaviours in relation to antecedents and consequences, and systematically monitor changes in behaviour as various empirical interventions are undertaken. This approach has led to the development of "positive behavioural support," which incorporates both the modification of the target behaviour and reinforcement of more adaptive behaviours to improve functioning and enhance communication.

For example, in 2007 McLean and colleagues reported an evaluation of positive behavioural support in providing care for five adults with developmental disabilities and severe aggressive behaviour in the community. The services included behavioural meetings with caregivers, mental health reviews, intensive support for direct care staff, emergency respite, and crisis response. Following intervention, significant improvements were reported for behaviour, quality of life, mental health, and medication use. Beyond the individuals themselves, environmental modifications were also considered including measures to reduce noise or avoid noisy environments.

Contemporary behaviour support plans include "proactive" and "reactive" strategies. The former strategies are directed at prevention and at the presumed setting/event/cause of the problem behaviour as identified in a functional assessment. For example, prevention might entail making changes to the person's environment or providing life skills training. Reactive strategies are designed to deal with the problem behaviour when it occurs, particularly to reduce any risk of harm to the individual or to the caregivers. Ideally, in treating behavioural features, relevant biomedical and behavioural interventions are provided together and in collaboration to maximize efficacy. Behaviour therapists normally work under the supervision of registered clinical psychologists who develop and monitor the behavioural interventions and support plans in line with the overall treatment-management plan.

Psychotherapy/Counselling

Psychotherapy and counselling, terms used interchangeably here, are relatively unrecognized and underutilized in the care of persons with developmental disabilities. Therapists "tailor" their approach to the individual; they establish a therapeutic alliance and professional relationship with the individual to identify, remove, or modify symptoms or patterns of behaviour while promoting personal growth and development.

Lynch (2004) observes that growing interest in these interventions reflects the willingness of therapists to modify traditional approaches, to overcome their own negative attitudes about these individuals, and to recognize the importance of involving caregivers in the treatment process. He lists strategies that are important in ensuring progress such as simplifying language, presenting information at a slower rate, checking for comprehension of concepts, using non-verbal communication, employing role-playing to bolster learning, and making concepts relevant to recent real-life situations.

In the UK, Lindsay and his colleagues have used group cognitive-behavioural models (including role-playing, progressive relaxation, visual imagery, and diaries) to treat irritability and aggression in individuals with mild to moderate developmental disabilities. And Nigel Beail, a UK psychologist, has shown that weekly "psychodynamic psychotherapy" sessions over several months have benefited males with mild intellectual disabilities and delinquent behaviours. It is noteworthy for clinicians, given the continuing care needs of this population, that ongoing supportive counselling (e.g., regular check-ins) can be very effective in preventing future crises not otherwise addressed in time-limited approaches.

UK psychiatrist Sheila Hollins has prepared a series of illustrated story books, *Beyond Words*, to foster and improve communication with individuals with intellectual disability; noteworthy examples include *Feeling Blue, Falling in Love, When Dad Died,* and *Getting on With Epilepsy.*

Finally, clinical psychologists in the UK receive subspecialty training in "learning disabilities" including experience with non-disabled individuals over the lifespan. Such training increases the awareness of all clinicians that they will be exposed to individuals with developmental disabilities and dual diagnosis irrespective of their chosen specialty after training.

In Canada, psychotherapy and counselling is provided by psychiatrists, clinical psychologists, and social workers, most of whom apply the principles and approaches they have learned in treating non-intellectually impaired individuals to those with developmental disabilities.

Rehabilitation Therapies

Implied in the term "rehabilitation therapy" is the restoration of functional abilities lost through illness rather than their promotion in an individual with developmental disability in whom they are yet to develop. This distinction is inherent in a 1990 book on "habilitation planning" for adults with disabilities by Schalock and Kiernan. They identify behavioural training technology, programmatic features of quality services, and quality-of-life program practices as important principles in serving this population.

Speech-language pathologists working with this population focus their efforts on improving language and enhancing communication skills with therapy and augmentative communication devices (e.g., choice boards, visual schedules, picture exchange systems) and on specific issues concerned with mastication and swallowing. They have a major role in conducting speech-language assessments and guiding communication disorder assistants or other caregivers in follow-up activities to improve communication through speech, sign, or visual programs.

Occupational therapists have a somewhat wider perspective, indeed beyond "occupation" or work, to promote optimal functioning in self-care and in various vocational and leisure activities. For individuals with autism spectrum disorders, occupational therapists also assess sensory integration disorders and develop related interventions (e.g., sensory diets). The role of physiotherapists is related to their knowledge and skills in the areas of mobility, stamina, and fitness. Physiotherapy is most relevant for individuals with cerebral palsy, ambulatory difficulties, and other "spasticity" concerns.

Any of the rehabilitation therapists may work directly with individuals with developmental disabilities, or they may assist indirectly through providing consultation to caregivers and education in the prescription of any "assistive devices" to enhance the environment. While training programs for rehabilitation therapists may have neglected the field of developmental disabilities and dual diagnosis, in particular adults, there is growing recognition that these disciplines make very significant contributions to "habilitation planning" and promoting optimal functioning in day-to-day living.

FURTHER READINGS:

Beail, N. (1998). Psychoanalytic psychotherapy with men with intellectual disabilities: a preliminary outcome study. *British Journal of Medical Psychology, 71*, 1-11.

Hollins, S., & Sinason, V. (2000). Psychotherapy, learning disabilities and trauma: New perspectives. *British Journal of Psychiatry, 176*, 320-336.

Lynch, C. (2004). Psychotherapy for persons with mental retardation. *Mental Retardation, 42*(5), 399-405.

McLean, B., Dench, C., & Grey, I., Shanahan, S., Fitzsimons, E., Hendler, J., & Corrigan, M. (2005). Person focused training: A model for delivering positive behaviour supports to people with challenging behaviours. *Journal of Intellectual Disability Research, 49*, 340-352.

Schalock, R., & Kiernan, W. (1990). *Habilitation planning for adults with disabilities.* New York: Springer-Verlag.

Willner, P., Jones, J., Tams, R., & Green, G. (2002). *A randomized controlled trial of the efficacy of a cognitive-behavioural anger management group for clients with learning disabilities.* Swansea, UK: Llwyneryr Unit, Department of Psychology, Bro Morgannwg NHS Trust.

2.4.3 Biomedical Treatments

Most biomedical treatments for persons with developmental disabilities are provided in the community. Occasionally, as outlined in Section 2.5, an interval of residential or hospital treatment is required to supplement community treatment. These arrangements provide opportunities for highly specialized assessments and intensive interventions that are not possible while the individual lives at home.

Biomedical treatments, medical and psychiatric, rely on traditional approaches to diagnosis and categorization of particular disorders. The aim is to identify causative factors and either modify their severity or, ideally, eliminate them and thereby relieve the individual's symptomatology. To this end a variety of diagnostic investigations including laboratory tests and imaging are followed by various treatments (e.g., diets, medications, surgery) that will disrupt the "disease process." These approaches have been most successful in illnesses like acute infections, and much less so with chronic illnesses and disabilities that have gradually become the focus of contemporary practice. It is in such situations that innovative approaches in healthcare delivery are desirable.

Medical Treatment

Medical treatment, although often overseen by a physician, is frequently provided by a team of professionals including nurse practitioners, nurses, pharmacists, and dietitians. Clinical practice guidelines have been prepared to ensure systematic use of evidence-based approaches to treatment; such guidelines are now available in Canada for individuals with developmental disabilities, although presently it is unclear as to the extent of their application in mainstream healthcare.

Since individuals with developmental disabilities are predisposed to certain disorders (see Section 1.4) and are less likely to recognize and report indicators of personal ill-health of any kind, monitoring and clinical vigilance by caregivers and healthcare professionals are extremely important issues. Lennox and his colleagues (2001) in Australia have created a clinical tool to engage caregivers and primary care providers in joint efforts to monitor health and foster health-promotion activities.

It is increasingly clear from studying the patterns of undetected morbidity and premature mortality in persons with developmental disabilities receiving mainstream healthcare that consultant specialists are needed in contemporary practice. This approach has been pioneered in the Netherlands and is being explored in the UK, with unfortunately little if any attention in Canada. Subspecialists are needed to train mainstream providers, to consult as needed in the care of those with particularly challenging circumstances, and to conduct research at both basic and applied levels. Although research on the medical problems of persons with developmental disabilities is scarce, those of us involved have concluded that generic provision is not sufficient to achieve equity in healthcare outcomes—equity in outcomes requires the provision of medical expertise beyond that set aside for the general population. Meanwhile, physicians, nurses, and other health professionals provide the best care they can without the benefits of consulting specialists.

Psychiatric Treatment

Psychiatric treatment for persons with developmental disabilities is obviously focused on the 30–40% with a dual diagnosis. Based on the individual's clinical history and a "mental status" examination, the psychiatrist prepares a diagnostic formulation and a treatment-management plan. Formulating a treatment-management plan is an interprofessional endeavour. Members of the mental health team may include clinical psychologists, social workers, nurses, and rehabilitation therapists. An interprofessional team approach is preferred for individuals with a dual diagnosis given their complex needs.

In the UK, "learning disabilities psychiatry" is a recognized psychiatric subspecialty. Training for these subspecialists, while including experience with individuals who do not have a developmental disability, is focused on the dual diagnosis population. Mainstream psychiatrists are encouraged to include individuals with dual diagnosis in their practices, often with consultative assistance from the subspecialists, but the subspecialist group provides most of the care for those with severe disabilities and complex health and mental health problems. They have made major scholarly contributions to the field of dual diagnosis, including DC-LD (described in Section 1.5) and the Frith Prescribing Guidelines for the use of psychotropic medications. Another subgroup has taken up the challenge of specialized training in psychotherapy for persons with developmental disabilities.

Canada has much to learn from the UK experience. Unfortunately, planners and educators here perseverate in thinking that persons with dual diagnosis can be managed completely by mainstream psychiatrists.

Further Readings:

Bhaumik, S., & Branford, D. (Eds.). (2005). *The Frith Prescribing Guidelines for adults with learning disability.* London: Taylor & Francis.

Lennox, N., Green, M., Diggens, J., & Ugoni, A. (2001). Audit and comprehensive health assessment programmes in the primary healthcare of adults with intellectual disability: A pilot study. *Journal of Intellectual Disability Research, 45*(3), 226-232.

2.5 To be familiar with the provision of residential and hospital treatment-management plans

As previously noted, sometimes an interval of treatment in a special residential or hospital setting is needed for an individual with a developmental disability. A person may be hospitalized for medical or surgical illnesses, dental care under anesthesia, and mental health crises. Such intervals contrast with life-long stays during the institutional era; today, the individual has a home in the community and will return there as soon as the problem prompting residential or hospital care is resolved.

Health professionals and caregivers should make every effort to ensure "continuity of care," even though residential and hospital treatment is often provided by professionals "new" to the individual. Clinical records in both community residential and hospital practices should reflect the needs of the individual and the caregivers for a smooth transition and transfer of clinical responsibility.

Unfortunately, in Canada, those responsible for planning a range of community residential options for persons with developmental disabilities have been preoccupied with creating "homes" and avoiding "treatment" options. Community and social service ministries focus on providing accommodation, leaving treatment options to the heathcare system; the result is a fragmented system of care. Clinical treatment for people with developmental disabilities and dual diagnosis in a specialized setting is seen as inconsistent with the principle of normalization whereby anyone, disabled or not, will be treated in a local hospital. This division of responsibilities has left many individuals and families without adequate care in the community.

2.5.1 Residential Treatment

If the range of community residential options is to include a setting for "residential treatment," its focus is clients with "challenging behaviours," ideally those whose behaviours are primary and not a manifestation of a medical or psychiatric illness. For such clients, functional assessment and intensive behaviour management are necessary, usually over several months, followed by a gradual reintegration to their permanent homes. Residential treatment is usually supervised by a registered clinical psychologist and provided by behavioural therapists and residential counsellors. Medical and psychiatric consultations are arranged as needed. While long-term use of antipsychotic medications for the treatment of problem behaviours is no longer defensible, other categories such as mood stabilizers, anticonvulsants, and propanolol are useful in selected cases of treating resistant aggression, and baclofen or naltrexone for self-injury.

2.5.2 Hospital Treatment

Admission for inpatient hospital treatment can occur on an emergency basis or on an elective basis. Emergency admissions reflect a very acute change in the individual's physical or mental state. This change is associated with a need for intensive treatment, often in a ward that can be locked under the terms of a province's mental health legislation. In contrast, elective admissions are indicated when community care is not proceeding satisfactorily and the professionals involved conclude that necessary treatment can be provided on an inpatient unit. Elective admissions may need to be involuntary, although most are negotiated on a voluntary basis with the individual and his or her substitute decision maker if necessary.

Acute Inpatient Treatment

Acute inpatient treatment appears to be most relevant for persons with mild intellectual impairment who are acutely psychotic, aggressive, or suicidal. Most psychiatric nurses, given that verbal communication is usually possible, are comfortable with these individuals. They should be asked to be vigilant for evidence of exploitation, intimidation, or abuse by other patients, particularly by those with personality disorders or histories of antisocial behaviour. Whenever possible, family members and caregivers from the social services sector who are acquainted with the individual should be consulted about his or her needs, vulnerabilities, and personal characteristics. These consultations foster not only optimal care during the admission but also smooth discharge and transition back to the community.

Studies on acute inpatient care reveal that the average duration of stay for individuals with dual diagnosis may be a few days beyond that observed for individuals without intellectual impairment. Outliers beyond a few days are often those whose residential arrangements prior to admission have failed, and social workers need more time to find suitable alternatives. Observations in the United Kingdom suggest that a general population of 100,000 implies a need for 1–2 acute inpatient beds for individuals with dual diagnosis.

Extended Inpatient Treatment

Extended inpatient treatment, often in a regional psychiatric hospital, appears to be most relevant for those with intellectual impairment whose dual diagnosis involves significant "behaviour management" challenges and treatment-resistant illness. Accordingly, the treatment program will normally focus exclusively on this population, and staffing should include both psychiatric nursing and behavioural therapists. Insofar as possible, admissions for extended treatment should be elective. The particular "targets" for resolution during the inpatient stay (e.g., self-injury, destructiveness) should be identified in advance and a clear understanding established with the agency providing support in the social services sector that once these targets are met, discharge will occur. This approach minimizes the risk of "silting up" (i.e., the prolonged stay on an extended treatment unit of individuals who need long-term residential care but whose target behavioural difficulties have already been resolved). Although the number of persons with more severe intellectual impairment is significantly less than the number with mild intellectual impairment, given an average length of stay of 10–12 months, a population of 100,000 needs 8–10 beds devoted to extended treatment.

Suicide Risks

Although the risk of suicide of persons with intellectual disabilities is only one third of that observed in the general population, the risk indicators are similar. Inpatient clinicians must be aware of more likely behavioural presentations as compared to self-reports of inner turmoil. Accordingly, admission for inpatient care is often required for those with mild intellectual impairment who

- are depressed
- express suicidal intent
- have made previous attempts
- have had close relatives die from suicide
- have been abused

Care on an inpatient basis is the same as the care provided for suicidal individuals who are free from intellectual impairment.

Conflict With the Law and Self-injury

Individuals with developmental disabilities who have been or are in conflict with the law can be successfully treated as inpatients, and there is no published evidence of an increased length of stay. Inpatient treatment for individuals with dual diagnosis usually focuses on high-risk problematic behaviours and may involve the use of isolation and control-and-restraint procedures to minimize harm to self or others. Severe self-injurious behaviour is more frequent in persons with more severe levels of intellectual impairment. Physical and/or mechanical restraints (e.g., helmets, mitts) to prevent head or eye injuries, in particular, may therefore be required for those in extended treatment inpatient units.

Further Readings:

Bailey, N. M., & Cooper, S. A. (1997). The current provision of specialist health services for people with learning disabilities. *Journal of Intellectual Disability Research, 41*(1), 52-59.

Chaplin, R. (2004). Review: General psychiatric services for adults with intellectual disability and mental illness. *Journal of Intellectual Disability Research, 48*(1), 1-10.

Gardner, W. I., & Hunter, R. H. (2003). Psychosocial diagnosis and treatment services in inpatient psychiatric facilities for persons with mental retardation. *Practice Guide Mental Health Aspects of Developmental Disability*, 6(2), 68-80.

Jones, J. (2007). Persons with intellectual disabilities in the criminal justice system: Review of issues. *International Journal of Offender Therapy and Comparative Criminology, 51*(6), 723.

Patja, K. (2004). Suicide cases in a population-based cohort of persons with intellectual disability in a 35 year follow-up. *Mental Health Aspects of Developmental Disability*, 7(4), 117-123.

Reed, S., Russell, A., Xenetidis, K., & Murphy, D. (2004). People with learning disabilities in a low secure inpatient unit: Comparison of offenders vs non-offenders. *British Journal of Psychiatry, 185*, 499-504.

PART 3 – ATTITUDES

Societal and professional attitudes about persons with developmental disabilities have a powerful and pervasive impact, often poorly understood, on quality of life for these individuals.

Societal attitudes, initially paternalistic protectiveness and later eugenic fears, fostered the role of institutions in the last century. Eugenic beliefs escalated in Nazi Germany during World War II resulting in involuntary sterilization of persons with intellectual disabilities and later their euthanasia. After World War II, a strong advocacy movement pressured for the closure of institutions and the promotion of a "normal" life in the community (i.e., normalization and social inclusion).

Professional attitudes reflect both societal attitudes and the evolution and standards of the various professional disciplines. Accordingly, in the subsections that follow, professional attitudes about individuals with developmental disabilities, caregivers, and interprofessional teamwork are considered. Next, the desirability of professional vigilance about vulnerability and the risk of abuse is outlined. Finally, the implications of reduced mental capacity on decision-making are discussed.

Unfortunately, it is difficult to avoid the conclusion that both societal and professional attitudes have often hindered, not helped, persons with developmental disabilities over the past century. It is to be hoped that their lot in life will improve in the 21st century, both in relation to general societal support and in the provision of adequate and respectful professional services.

FURTHER READING:

Shakespeare, T., & Grace, N. E. (2009). Disability and the training of health professionals. *Lancet, 374*, 1815-1816.

3.1 To develop empathetic awareness of the special needs of persons with developmental disabilities and dual diagnosis for respectful health and mental healthcare

In 1998 Jean Vanier, the Canadian who founded the L'Arche organization, described individuals with intellectual disabilities as "among the most oppressed and excluded people in the world." While Vanier may not have been referring specifically to healthcare professionals, unfortunately there is clear and continuing evidence of indifference to the special needs of this population and neglect of the topic in professional healthcare training programs. Consideration of this indifference and neglect is the focus of this section.

In most Canadian provinces, the agencies primarily responsible for supporting persons with developmental disabilities are funded as "social services," not "health services." The true "social cost" of developmental disabilities includes people's needs for both social support and healthcare. Some insight about these matters is provided in a 2002 report from the Netherlands by Polder, Meerding, Bonneux, and VanderMass; they concluded that 9% of health spending was directed at intellectual disabilities. A comparable investigation is needed in Canada to ensure that some of the indifference to the special needs of persons with developmental disabilities is not based simply on a failure to recognize just how costly these healthcare needs can be, including the additional costs involved in poor interministerial and interagency coordination of effort.

Although there is a relatively small literature on the inclusion of the field of intellectual disability in training programs for healthcare professionals, observations published on training psychiatrists suggest the topic is often neglected. As far back as 1965, American psychiatrist Howard Potter described "mental retardation" as the "Cinderella of Psychiatry." He strongly recommended enhanced training for medical students and psychiatry residents so that the service challenges of the era could be addressed. Surveys of psychiatry training programs in Canada have consistently revealed inadequate levels of instruction, and the most recent study by Lunsky and Bradley (2001) concluded that the situation is deteriorating, not improving. It seems clear that the almost total neglect of intellectual disability in psychiatry training programs can explain the indifference to the needs of the population observed in mental health services. Were anxiety disorders or schizophrenia similarly neglected, comparable indifference to these individuals would be expected.

The situation of educational neglect and insufficient training in developmental disabilities is similar across other healthcare professions (e.g., psychology, rehabilitation therapy, and social work). Subspecialty training is nonexistent, although some disciplines receive exposure to child-related issues in pediatrics and developmental psychology.

Over the past decade in the UK, the neglect of the special healthcare needs of persons with intellectual disabilities has been exposed by MENCAP. A national advocacy organization, MENCAP launched a campaign ("Treat Me Right") for improved health services for persons with "learning disabilities" in 2004. Then in 2007, the organization published *Death by Indifference*, a report on the unfortunate circumstances surrounding the premature deaths of six individuals with learning disabilities. Therein MENCAP alleged that the

National Health Service displayed "institutional discrimination" against these individuals. As evidence, the report listed a number of key factors involved:

- People with a learning disability are seen to be a low priority.
- Many healthcare professionals do not understand enough about learning disabilities.
- Many healthcare professionals do not properly consult and involve families and carers of people with a learning disability.
- Many healthcare professionals do not understand the law around capacity and consent to treatment.
- Healthcare professionals rely inappropriately on their estimates of a person's quality of life.

Death by Indifference was followed in 2008 by a major review of these issues and a set of broad-ranging recommendations to remedy the situation. The recommendation included better training for healthcare professionals and annual health checks for individuals with intellectual disabilities by their primary care providers. Such measures could usefully be implemented in Canada.

There is a moral issue implied in the contemporary indifference to the needs of this population and neglect of the topic in professional healthcare training programs. The Nazi era in Germany in the last century illustrates how easily indifference and neglect can give way to things far more "evil." There is ample evidence that German physicians were intimately involved in the selection of those with mental retardation, often living in institutions, for involuntary surgical sterilization and later for death. Training programs should therefore be reviewed and revised to address the needs of even those with the most severe levels of intellectual impairment. Although the language might be outdated, Lionel Penrose eloquently describes the needs of this group in *The Biology of Mental Defect*, published in 1963:

> Not only are these low-grade defectives harmless, they are not responsible for their own condition. They can be happy and they can stimulate human feelings and parental love. By all canons of civilized society, they have a right to demand care and comfort even if they are unable to give adequate returns. The ability of a community to make satisfactory provision for its defectives is an index of its own health and progressive development. The desire for their euthanasia is a sign of involution and decay of human standards. (pp. 292-293)

There is a large gap between the expectations articulated by Penrose and the oppression and exclusion noted more recently by Jean Vanier. To close it, healthcare training programs must be improved to equip graduates to provide expertise and to work productively with others in serving those with developmental disabilities and dual diagnosis.

FURTHER READINGS:

Lifton, R. J. (1986). *Medical killing and the psychology of genocide: The Nazi doctors.* New York: Basic Books.

Lunsky, Y., & Bradley, E. (2001). Developmental disabilities in Canadian psychiatry residency programs. *Canadian Journal of Psychiatry, 46,* 138-143.

MENCAP. (2007). *Death by indifference.* www.mencap.org.uk

Penrose, L. S. (1963). *The biology of mental defect.* London: Sidgwich and Jackson.

Polder, J. J., Meerding, W. J., Bonneux, L., & VanderMaas, P. J. (2002). Healthcare costs of intellectual disability in the Netherlands: A cost of illness perspective. *Journal of Intellectual Disability Research, 46*(2), 168-178.

Potter, H. W. (1965). Mental retardation: The Cinderella of psychiatry. *Psychiatric Quarterly, 39,* 537-549.

3.2 To identify with the challenges experienced by family and agency caregivers who provide care and support for persons with developmental disabilities and dual diagnosis

Although adults with developmental disabilities are best thought of as adults with special needs, the concept of the "eternal child" is a reminder that they often need lifelong support. The burden of care is shared by different caregivers in a pattern that is primarily parental in childhood and primarily protective and assumed by agency staff in later years. This subsection discusses the underlying attitudes that will help healthcare professionals to cultivate positive relationships with caregivers over the individual's lifespan.

Parents of young children with disabilities frequently refer to the "daily grind" when they describe life with a child who is significantly slow in reaching developmental milestones. Clinicians should acknowledge their commitment and hard work. Fatigue is inevitable, and so clinicians should encourage parents to take regular breaks, pointing out that any guilt that parents might feel is outweighed by the benefits of respite for all concerned. Those with financial problems should be informed of the availability of children's disability allowances, designed to pay for assistive devices, diets, and respite care. Clinicians who are optimistic and respectful, and who provide advice about available supports are an asset in helping young families get through the challenging period from diagnosis to ongoing support and daily care.

Parents of school-aged children with disabilities face some "new" stressors, such as how the children are educated and cared for in schools, daycare settings, and summer camps. Concerns tend to escalate in the "transitional" years given physical and sexual maturation, aspirations of independence, and the usual risk of substance abuse and the "testing" adult social roles. Professionals need to understand these developments, and to provide advice and guidance about these challenges for parents as they occur. At the same time, healthcare professionals must collaborate with social service providers who will play an important role in helping the individual become more independent.

Although the benefits may not be immediately obvious, it is likely optimal for both the individual and family that the person with disabilities move to new accommodation in early adulthood. This transition can foster independence. It also averts the unfortunate scenario where the "eternal child" stays on with the parents until parental illness or death renders a move absolutely necessary. On occasion, this means that professionals will need to discuss a move to adult service somewhat before the parents may be psychologically or emotionally ready for such a move. Counselling for parents along these lines is especially difficult because in many jurisdictions planners have little if any idea what the projected caseload for adult services might be, and seemingly impossible waiting lists for service exist. This neglectful societal attitude need not be supported by professional consultants whose concerns for individuals with developmental disabilities and family caregivers should override bureaucratic ineptitude. In Section 3.3 the important role of regional case registers in facilitating optimal planning is reviewed.

Some adults with developmental disabilities are not capable of making independent decisions. If they are placed in a residential program, a parent or sibling will usually have a continuing legal role as a substitute decision maker for personal and financial matters. Sometimes, a clinician will become aware of conflicting opinions about treatment among family and agency caregivers. The clinician can help to negotiate a consensus by focusing on the "best interests" of the individual and quality of life, while respecting the differing perspectives.

Finally, there are situations where the focus of concern is on agency caregivers alone. Included here are misunderstandings about the goals of treatment, conflicting perspectives between staff members within the agency itself, staff burnout, and rapid staff turnover. Healthcare professionals, while vigilant about the impact of these problems on their client with developmental disabilities, also need to respect the role of the management of the agency in resolving them. Insofar as possible, unless there is evidence of serious mistreatment, clinicians should identify and discuss these matters with the individual and the accompanying caregiver. The discussion will be reflected in the progress note outlining the visit. If the clinician is consulted later by agency managers, the progress note will be a useful point of reference. Issues of suspected abuse require additional steps, as outlined in Section 3.4.

Further Readings:

Barron, A., & Hassiotis, A. (2008). Good practice in transition services for young people with learning disabilities: A review. *Advances in Mental Health and Learning Disabilities, 2*(3), 18-22.

Minnes, P., & Burbidge, J. (2012). Family life and developmental disability. In I. Brown & M. Percy (Eds.), *Developmental disabilities in Ontario* (3rd ed., pp. 851-872). Toronto: Ontario Association on Developmental Disabilities.

3.3 To respect the contributions of various professional disciplines who provide services for persons with developmental disabilities and dual diagnosis

This section is concerned with attitudes that influence the function of interprofessional teams and the collaborative roles of team members. Collaboration is important, because people with developmental disabilities have complex needs. Coordinated interdisciplinary and cross-sector efforts are required to meet those needs.

Professionals involved in the field of developmental disabilities are often asked by colleagues from other disciplines to define their particular contributions to care. Such requests appear to reflect a general lack of knowledge about developmental disabilities and about the need for collaborative interprofessional efforts in providing care. Neglect of developmental disabilities in professional training programs can be ascribed to societal attitudes about these individuals, as well as a dearth of faculty who themselves have expertise in the field. During the institutional era of care, professional training occurred "on the job." Community care requires "new" knowledge, skills, and attitudes and, to date, such training is inconsistently available or inadequately applied.

Developmental disabilities, heterogeneous in origin and homogeneous only in sharing lifelong cognitive and adaptive problems, are not primarily medical or educational or social disorders. Rather, they are all of these at one time or another, sometimes all at once! None of the professionals from these three sectors can claim a monopoly on providing care. In fact, none of the various professional disciplines gives developmental disabilities adequate attention, either in professional training or in research. All of these factors influence the operation of interprofessional teams assigned to closing institutions and providing optimal care in the community. Apart from the goal of "social inclusion," there is little to foster effective collaboration beyond the collective goodwill of the team members themselves.

Although the institutional era can now be said to be over, a blueprint for successful community care is far from complete. Professional goodwill can catalyze innovations that are obviously needed. Collectively, team members need to recognize how to overcome the shortcomings in their training about developmental disabilities, and to learn from each other and from individuals with disabilities. They need to respect the history and conceptual frameworks that underlie each professional discipline, and to avoid the risks associated with traditional hierarchies and power structures. And they need to learn about the value of research in moving forward the agenda of optimal community care, be this basic research or applied.

Early in the 21st century it has become obvious that a major roadblock in providing a blueprint for successful community care is the "silo" attitude that prevents interprofessional training and research. While there may be funds for healthcare, education, or social services, there is little shared funding and minimal attention to funding training and research about cross-sectoral collaboration. Accordingly, those professionals who have found their way into the interprofessional enterprise on behalf of persons with developmental disabilities must recognize that their collaborative teamwork may itself be the key to developing necessary insights about community care.

A regional case register can be an invaluable tool in promoting cross-sectoral collaboration in serving all the individuals from a region requiring care because of a developmental disability. Although some case registers focus on adults only, ideally a child is listed on the register when the developmental disability is first identified and remains there through the transition to adulthood and beyond. Professionals and agencies from all sectors are provided with information important for planning for individuals or groups. Forecasting caseloads and human resource requirements is critically important as the individuals from the region mature and life situations evolve. Case register data can be useful in training students and researchers in the field of developmental disabilities. It should not be surprising to learn that case registers already exist in many jurisdictions that have closed their institutions and now rely on interprofessional teams to provide comprehensive and collaborative community care.

It is suggested here that insights are emerging from professionals who provide interprofessional, collaborative care in the community. These insights lead to the development of useful tools, like a regional case register. Indeed, in the absence of such tools, it seems likely the unfortunate "silo" attitude and related policies will persist.

Further Reading:

Summers, J., Boyd, K., & Reid, J., Adamson, J., Habjan, B., Gignae, V., & Moister, C. (2002). The interdisciplinary mental health team. In D. M. Griffiths, C. Stavrakaki, & J. Summers (Eds.), *Dual diagnosis: An introduction to the mental health needs of persons with developmental disabilities* (pp. 325-358). Sudbury: Habilitative Mental Health Resource Network.

3.4 To develop vigilance regarding the risk of neglect and abuse observed in persons with developmental disabilities and dual diagnosis

Section 3.1 discussed the historical maltreatment of persons with developmental disabilities, escalating to widespread euthanasia in Nazi Germany. This section considers the neglect and abuse that healthcare professionals may observe in contemporary practice, and how they should respond.

As institutions are decommissioned and as a policy of social inclusion is implemented, it is becoming obvious that such inclusion is rarely automatic. Simply providing a place to live in the community does not mean that inclusion in mainstream education, health, and social services will follow. And when it does not occur, individuals with developmental disabilities and, indirectly, their families and caregivers, are experiencing the effects of neglect. In these circumstances, healthcare providers may observe individuals who are demoralized, depressed, or "acting out" their challenges, and caregivers who are frustrated and overburdened in carrying out their responsibilities.

The true social cost of deinstitutionalization will gradually emerge as the advocates who promoted it as a better and cheaper approach to care are replaced by a new generation of advocates who are addressing contemporary neglect and fiscal need. Unfortunately, unlike in the UK where MENCAP advocates for all citizens with developmental disabilities, there is no national counterpart in Canada. Apart from some recent efforts to see persons with dual diagnosis included in "chronic care" advocacy for mental health reform in Canada, there appears to be little immediate chance of forming a credible advocacy organization.

In these circumstances, what can practicing healthcare professionals contribute? In the first instance, they should be vigilant about the effects of neglect when evaluating individuals with developmental disabilities. Second, healthcare professionals can adjust their own practices to ensure inclusion; such adjustments will take time and effort, however, that are unlikely to be recognized in current fee schedules and service structures. Finally, healthcare professionals can use their good offices to write letters of support for individuals who are applying for funds to enhance care in their community.

Any evidence that an adult with developmental disabilities might have experienced physical or sexual assault demands immediate clinical attention, although there are no regulations like "child welfare" legislation for adults. Persons with developmental disabilities who cannot take themselves out of a situation or voice a complaint are particularly vulnerable. Appropriate examination and documentation are needed. Normally, police and the relevant authorities should be called, particularly if the caregiver or an agency is thought to be the alleged offender. Obviously these are complex and potentially controversial situations, but a professional's "duty to care" can support the approach outlined here. Ruth Ryan, an American psychiatrist who specializes in the care of persons with developmental disabilities, has made a number of practical suggestions. She recommends that neglect or abuse be considered if a person's level of adjustment deteriorates. She regards home visits by a member of the clinic team to be essential, and also suggests that a "behaviour support" service referral should precede orders for restraint, seclusion, or PRN sedation.

FURTHER READING:

Ryan, R. (2001). Physician unwitting participation in abuse and neglect of persons with developmental disabilities. *Community Mental Health Journal, 37*(6), 499-509.

3.5 To acknowledge important attitudinal variables involved in providing optimal care and support for individuals with reduced mental capacity to make decisions

While severe levels of intellectual impairment are more likely associated with reduced "mental capacity," many with mild intellectual impairment, particularly as adults, can learn to make reasonable decisions. Accordingly, like some individuals with dementia, only some individuals with developmental disabilities can be said to have functionally significant reductions in mental capacity. In practice, this means that healthcare professionals have to treat each individual and each situation separately. Situations where issues of mental capacity are relevant include consent to treatment, sexual expression, parenting, and conflict with the law.

It is the clinician's responsibility to determine whether an individual has the mental capacity to make informed decisions. Factors to consider are the person's ability to understand and retain relevant information, to appreciate how the information applies to him or her, to weigh the risks and benefits of a decision and alternatives, and to communicate the decision. Given that many individuals with intellectual disabilities come to depend on others for help in making decisions, it is always important to assess the degree to which the individual might feel inclined to acquiesce or follow advice rather than coming to an independent conclusion. When a clinician concludes that an individual is unable to provide informed consent, the law of the province will identify the closest relative or appoint a "public guardian" who is authorized to serve as a "substitute decision maker" and to act in the individual's "best interest."

Since 1986, when the Supreme Court of Canada decided that the mother of a woman with developmental disabilities (i.e., The Eve case) could not provide substitute consent for a surgical sterilization, there have been no permanent legal methods to limit reproduction in such circumstances; otherwise any necessary "treatments" can be provided. For persons with a dual diagnosis, provincial mental health legislation is applied in the usual fashion, including "community treatment orders" and involuntary hospital admissions.

Sexual expression by persons with developmental disabilities has been poorly accepted and understood, and ignorance about it is associated with anxiety and unfortunate overreaction. Traditional institutions during the eugenic era segregated males and females, thereby promoting secretive heterosexual relationships and "situational" homosexuality. Masturbation was also discouraged because it was thought to be harmful. In contemporary society, although respect for sexual expression has improved, many caregivers are uncomfortable and at best apprehensive in dealing with the issues. There is vigilance that females not "be taken advantage of" by assertive males, a difficult scenario especially for those women with mild intellectual impairment who seek out attention and affection, and sometimes desire a pregnancy. Males may engage in sexually inappropriate behaviour or sexual exploration of children of either gender, a situation called "counterfeit deviance" to distinguish it from much less common paraphilia.

When a clinician is consulted about these matters, there is usually a halo of anxiety and uncertainty around caregivers and of frustration and guilt around the individual with a developmental disability. The history and examination may reveal not only reduced mental capacity but also evidence that the individual's need for social-sexual education and sexuality guidance has been somewhat neglected. In these circumstances, "treatment" for the individual usually consists of psychotherapy directed at validating sexual desires and reducing guilt and frustration. Counselling obviously needs to be folded into a management plan that combines sex education and some degree of personal supervision. The level of supervision will lessen as the individual's social judgment matures and "socially appropriate" behaviour increases.

For persons with reduced mental capacity who gradually learn to live with minimal supervision in the community, the desire to be "normal like everyone else" and, therefore, start a family can be a major concern to caregivers. But each case must be examined carefully—long gone is the era when involuntary sterilization was the "solution" for all concerned. The female involved is the focus of the assessment, but a competent and supportive partner and the availability of an extended family that can help may make a significant difference. When a couple does start a family, community support services like parent-child support groups and preschool nurseries can also be engaged to assist. Perhaps the most useful index of parenting capacity is what evolves after the fact, with respect to the first child. Child welfare authorities can be engaged at any stage and must be called in the event of significant neglect or abuse of any child, an obligation set out clearly in contemporary child welfare legislation and individual professional regulations.

Clinicians may be asked by legal counsel to assess an individual with a developmental disability who is "in conflict with the law." In these cases, the person's intellectual impairment may be an important factor in the evaluation of the offending behaviour and disposition of any criminal charges that have been laid. In conducting an assessment, the clinician should ask the lawyer to set out in writing the "facts" of the case and to specify the kinds of questions that should be addressed in the professional report. As well, the clinician's report should consider the individual's insight and awareness that the behavioural incident was against the law, and the natural inclination among those with developmental disabilities to answer "yes" to all questions. This tendency to acquiesce could affect what the individual has told police. Cognitive limitations that preclude "fitness to stand trial" or an inability to instruct counsel and follow court proceedings need to be identified before criminal responsibility is considered and evaluated.

Although the police, crown attorneys, and the judiciary have a duty to protect society, they are usually sensitive to the vulnerabilities and hazards that exist for persons with reduced mental capacity in these situations. They and the individual's defense attorney will take quite seriously any suggestions and recommendations put forth by mental health professionals for disposition so that persons with developmental disabilities, now free from incarceration in one sort of institution, do not find themselves locked up in another (i.e., so-called criminalization of the mentally ill).

Further Readings:

Griffiths, D. (2003). Sexuality of people who have developmental disabilities: From myth to emerging practices. In I. Brown & M. Percy (Eds.), *Developmental disabilities in Ontario* (2nd ed., pp. 677-690). Toronto: Ontario Association on Developmental Disabilities.

IASSID Special Interest Research Group on Parents and Parenting with Intellectual Disabilities. (2008). Parents labeled with intellectual disabilities: Position of IASSID SIRG on parents and parenting with intellectual disabilities. *Journal of Applied Research in Intellectual Disabilities, 21*, 296-307.

McCreary, B. D., & Thompson, J. (1999). Psychiatric aspects of sexual abuse involving persons with developmental disabilities. *Canadian Journal of Psychiatry, 44*, 350-355.

Peppin, P. (2002). Legal issues and ethical dimensions in dual diagnosis. In D. M. Griffiths, C. Stavrakaki, & J. Summers (Eds.), *Dual diagnosis: An introduction to the mental health needs of persons with developmental disabilities* (pp. 561-594). Sudbury, ON: Habilitative Mental Health Resource Network.

APPENDIX A
A Format for Recording the Clinical History

Date: ____________________________

I. **Patient**

Name: Address:

Date of birth:

Gender:

Allergies: Phone:

II. **Medical Care**

Health card number:

Family physician:

Address:

Phone:

III. **Next of Kin**

Name:

Relationship:

Address:

Phone:

IV. **Substitute Decision Maker**

Name:

Relationship:

Address:

Phone:

V. **Primary Support Agency** (developmental, mental health)

Name:

Address:

Phone:

VI. **Informant/Primary Support Worker**

Name:

Address:

Phone:

Presenting Concerns

I. Chief complaint (describe in 2-3 sentences)

II. Onset (when problem started, re-emerged or escalated to intolerable level)

III. "Stressors" at onset

- Biomedical (e.g., accidents, injuries, drug changes, decompensation of chronic illness)

- Psychosocial (e.g., bereavement, abuse, interpersonal conflict)

IV. Management/treatment to date

- Current medications (distinguish regular and PRN medications)

- Other interventions (hospitalized, respite care, police involved)

V. Change since onset (same, worsening, improving, new symptoms, medication side effects)

Patient Profile

I. Level of intellectual impairment (mild, moderate, severe, profound)

II. Level of adaptive behaviour (self-care, communication, literacy, job, family responsibility)

III. Residential supports (independent, supported independent living, group home, host family)

IV. Day programs and occupation

V. Key relationships (include partners and children if any)

VI. Sexual orientation and expression

VII. Personal interests and goals

VIII. Spiritual life

IX. Impression of contentment with present life situation

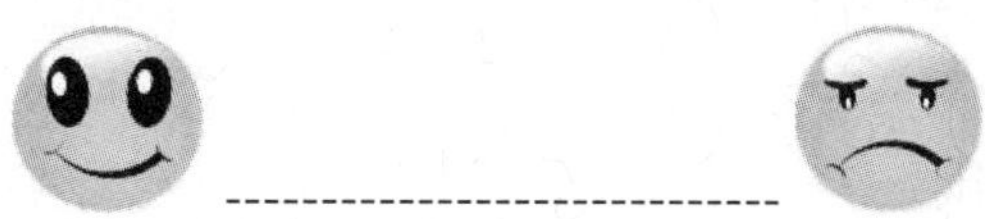

Biological** Family History

I. Father's Name:
   Age/age deceased:
   Occupation:
   Health/mental health:
   Cause of death:

II. Father's Family:
   Note relatives with developmental disability and mental disorders

III. Mother's Name:
   Age/age deceased:
   Occupation:
   Health/mental health:
   Cause of death:

IV. Mother's Family:
   Note relatives with developmental disability and mental disorders

V. Siblings*: (mother's pregnancies in chronological order, including abortions, miscarriages, and stillbirths)

   1.
   2.
   3.
   4.
   5.
   6.

   Continue on reverse side if needed
   *For each sibling: gender, age/age deceased, occupation, health/mental health, and cause of death

VI. 1. Are parents blood relatives? Yes No

   2. Are biological parents the main caregivers? Yes No
      If no, who are main caregivers?

   3. Have parents/family had genetics consultation/testing? Yes No
      If yes, where, when, results if known.

**Note: For individuals who are adopted/fostered:

Age of adoption/fostering:

Place of adoption/fostering:

Adoptive Father
Age/age deceased:
Occupation:
Health/mental health:
Cause of death:

Adoptive Mother
Age/age deceased:
Occupation:
Health/mental health:
Cause of death:

Developmental History

I. Prenatal development (infections, smoking, alcohol, medications, toxemia, hemorrhage)

II. Perinatal development (duration of pregnancy, birth weight, delivery, adjustment in neonatal period)

III. Postnatal development (illness, accidents, relationships with adults and peer groups)

IV. Developmental milestones
Social smile _____, sitting unsupported _____, crawling _____, walking _____, first words _____, speaking in sentences _____, bladder control _____, bowel control _____, nighttime continence _____.

V. Clinic contacts, hospitalizations in childhood

1.
2.
3.

Continue on reverse if needed

VI. School progress (mainstream, integrated, modified)
If "identified", when and in what category?
What accommodations recommended?

VII. Occupation and training (work history/income support/disability pension)

Health and Mental Health

I. List medical diagnoses (include congenital anomalies, sensory impairments, motor impairments, seizure disorders)

II. List psychiatric diagnosis (include childhood and adult disorders)

III. List hospital, clinic contacts (to facilitate transfer of records)

IV. Psychotropic drugs (include past and present)

V. Diet, nutrition, etc. (include special diets and food intolerance)

VI. Assistive devices (functional or communication)

VII. Conflict with the law (warnings, arrest, charges, convictions)
If a past victim, identify offending behaviour (e.g., sexual, physical, financial)

APPENDIX B

A Framework for Treatment-Management Planning

Name: ______________________ Date: ____________

Projected Review Date: ____________

Advocate: ____________________________________

<table>
<tr><th colspan="2">I. ASSESSMENT SUMMARY</th></tr>
<tr><td colspan="2">Clinical Summary</td></tr>
<tr><td colspan="2">DC/LD Summary</td></tr>
<tr><td colspan="2">Axis I Level of Intellectual Impairment</td></tr>
<tr><td colspan="2">Axis II Causes of Intellectual Impairment</td></tr>
<tr><td colspan="2">Axis III Level of Psychiatric Disorder</td></tr>
<tr><td>Level ____</td><td>Diagnosis ______________________</td></tr>
<tr><td></td><td>Biologic factors</td></tr>
<tr><td></td><td>Psychologic factors</td></tr>
<tr><td></td><td>Social factors</td></tr>
<tr><td></td><td>Developmental factors</td></tr>
<tr><td>Level ____</td><td>Diagnosis ______________________</td></tr>
<tr><td></td><td>Biologic factors</td></tr>
<tr><td></td><td>Psychologic factors</td></tr>
<tr><td></td><td>Social factors</td></tr>
<tr><td></td><td>Developmental factors</td></tr>
<tr><td>Health Problems:</td><td>Resiliency Issues:</td></tr>
<tr><td colspan="2">Prognostic Factors:</td></tr>
</table>

II. TREATMENT-MANAGEMENT PLAN
Developmental Services
◦ A place to live
◦ Meaningful occupation/activities
◦ Caregiver support and respite
Psychosocial Treatments
◦ Behaviour management
◦ Counselling/Psychotherapy
◦ Rehabilitation therapy
Biomedical Treatments
◦ Medical treatment
◦ Psychiatric treatment
◦ Residential or hospital treatment

APPENDIX C
SELF-EXAMINATION QUESTIONS AND ANSWERS

Exercise 1: True or False

1. Fragile X syndrome is a tri nucleotide repeat disorder.
2. Permanency planning is focused on moving from "education" to "life-skills" and vocational training.
3. Persons with cerebral palsy are always intellectually disabled.
4. Individuals with velocardiofacial syndrome are predisposed to schizophrenia.
5. Rett syndrome is linked to a mutation in the MECP2 gene located on the X chromosome.
6. Autism spectrum disorders are characterized by a triad of impairments in social interaction, communication, and imagination.
7. Phenylketonuria is a chromosome disorder.
8. Leo Kanner first described "autistic disturbances and affective content" in 1993.
9. Aggressive behaviour is linked to female gender.
10. Asperger syndrome is linked to male gender.
11. Pica is common in persons with mild intellectual disability.
12. The peak prevalence of mild intellectual disability occurs at age 12.
13. Permanency planning is focused on making plans for a person with developmental disabilities after the parents are deceased.
14. A parent with mild intellectual impairment can never raise a child successfully.
15. DC-LD is based on modifications of DSM-IV.

Exercise 1: Answers

1. True
2. False
3. False
4. True
5. True
6. True
7. False
8. False
9. True
10. True
11. False
12. True
13. True
14. False
15. False

Exercise 2: Multiple Choice

1. An individual with IQ scores ranging between 68 and 75 would be assumed to be capable of:

   a) holding an unskilled job
   b) obtaining basic literacy and numeracy skills
   c) serving as a juror
   d) completing Grade 5 in primary school
   e) serving in the military

2. Individuals with Down syndrome are somewhat predisposed to:

   a) obstructive sleep apnea
   b) hypothyroidism
   c) depression
   d) arteriosclerotic dementia
   e) Alzheimer's dementia

3. "Transition planning" is concerned with:

   a) leaving school and joining the workforce
   b) arrangements for guardianship following the parents' death
   c) leaving home and living in a community residence
   d) primary medical care from a family physician or nurse practitioner
   e) application for a disability pension

4. Pervasive developmental disorders can be associated with:

   a) Fragile X syndrome
   b) thimerosal-containing vaccines
   c) a mutation of the mecp2 gene on xq28
   d) tuberous sclerosis
   e) encephalitis

5. Anxiety symptoms are particularly common in:

   a) Down syndrome
   b) Williams syndrome
   c) velocardiofacial syndrome
   d) tuberous sclerosis
   e) Prader Willi syndrome

6. The central issue in The Eve case considered by the Supreme Court in 1986 was:

   a) fitness to stand trial
   b) the provision of a substitute consent for surgical sterilization
   c) parental neglect
   d) consent for ECT
   e) the relevance of a community treatment order

Exercise 2: Answers

1. a, b, and d
2. a, b, c, and e
3. a, c, d, and e
4. a, c, and d
5. b
6. b

APPENDIX D

CASE VIGNETTES

Preparation of assessment and treatment-management plans

This appendix provides an opportunity for the reader to apply what has been learned by creating treatment-management plans for five individuals with developmental disabilities described in the following vignettes. Readers should follow the format outlined in Appendix B to draft their plans, and compare them with the plans provided.

Clinical Summaries

Jesse

According to her group home counsellor, Jesse, a 51-year-old with Down syndrome, has become less sociable, apathetic, and occasionally "confused" over the past 5 months. The counsellor reports that when given a "three-step" task, Jesse can complete the first step successfully and then loses track of what to do next. The supervisor of the day program confirms the presence of these changes in behaviour.

Ed

Apart from earning small amounts of money doing manual odd jobs, Ed (age 21, diagnosed with mild intellectual disability at age 10), has been dependent on social welfare since he left a high school "special education" program 2 years ago. He lives with his mother, who now brings him to the emergency clinic after a violent aggressive incident at home the preceding evening. He tells you he has been hearing voices warning him he will lose his financial support and that his mother is going to kick him out of the house.

John

A father requests an urgent consultation at the clinic about his son John, a 17-year-old with moderate intellectual disabilities. John's parents have just been informed by a local police officer that John must respond to several complaints by neighbourhood parents that he engages in "sexual play" with younger children in the local park. If a formal complaint is received, the officer will find it necessary to lay a charge.

Ted

Ted is 20 and presents with depression. You learn that an assessment at age 12 revealed borderline intellectual functioning and Asperger syndrome. Now he has finished high school and plans to attend a community college to study computer technology. His mother, with whom he lives, reports he is anxious about his ability to relate to faculty and fellow students at the college. Ted says he is very worried and has contemplated suicide.

Sherri

Now 25, Sherri has engaged in self-injurious behaviour (SIB)—episodic head banging—since mid-childhood. She has a severe intellectual disability and a left hemiplegia. She is mobile in a wheelchair, has learned how to transfer, and attends a life-skills day program each morning. Her mother brought Sherri to the clinic because the current episode of SIB has been going on for 3 weeks and, unlike previous episodes which ended spontaneously, appears to be getting worse. There is bruising around Sherri's right eye.

Assessment for "Jesse"

DC-LD Summary

Axis I Unspecified intellectual disability

Axis II Down syndrome

Axis III Dementia, etiology not determined

- Biologic factors: predispositions to depression, sleep apnea, hypothyroidism and to Alzheimer's neuropathology
- Psychologic factors: possible symptomatic depressive syndrome
- Social factors: no apparent problems
- Developmental factors: pre-existing intellectual impairment distorts features of early dementia

Health Problems

- Review recent medical assessments and update as necessary, especially thyroid function
- Review past history for evidence of depressive episodes, obstructive sleep apnea

Resiliency Issues

- Maintain usual social contacts and daily and weekly routines
- Monitor appetite and weight

Treatment-Management Plan for "Jesse"

Developmental Services

- A place to live: maintain group home placement
- Meaningful activities: maintain day program and related recreational activities
- Caregiver support and respite: keep caregivers updated on results of further assessments and encourage continuity of care and respite

Psychosocial Treatment

- Behaviour management: complete "baseline" assessment of adaptive behaviour, social skills, mood, etc.
- Psychological assessment for baseline cognitive functioning screening for dementia and future comparative testing
- Counselling/Psychotherapy: not apparently relevant at this time

- Rehabilitation therapy: OT assessment to focus on current residential care and day program and to provide anticipatory guidance to caregivers regarding functional life skills (e.g., self-care, safety)

Biomedical Treatment

- Medical treatment: establish working diagnosis and treatment implications (including thyroid, mood, dementia, seizures)
- Psychiatric treatment: consultation for primary care provider and caregivers focused on diagnosis, prognosis, and medications (for hypothyroidism, depression, seizures, Alzheimer's dementia)
- Residential/hospital treatment: may become relevant if dementia progresses and precludes optimal care in the community, explore "nursing home" options as needed

Prognosis

- Alzheimer's dementia progresses to death from pneumonia over 5-year interval
- Hypothyroidism, depression, and seizures are treated symptomatically and usually successfully

Assessment for "Ed"

DC-LD Summary

Axis I Mild intellectual disability

Axis II Unspecified etiology

Axis III Level B, possible schizoaffective psychosis

- Biologic factors: screen for substance abuse, velocardiofacial syndrome
- Psychologic factors: investigate for "stressors" including peer group pressures (teasing, intimidation, abuse) and adjustment difficulties associated with transitional issues
- Social factors: review support available from family and developmental service agencies
- Developmental factors: pre-existing intellectual impairment implies special care in differential diagnosis and reaching working diagnosis, and poorer prognosis for full recovery

Health Problems

- Review recent medical assessments and update as necessary (e.g., toxic screen, CT scan, genetic testing)

Resiliency Issues

- Explore options for interpersonal relationships and for social and recreational pursuits
- Explore goals and expectations for future (both with individual and family)

Treatment-Management Plan for "Ed"

Developmental Services

- A place to live: if continued living with mother is problematic, arrange for suitability assessment supported-independent living (SIL) program e.g., apartment or suitable host family
- Meaningful activities: aim for optimal vocational options (e.g., community college) and social/recreational outlets. Stable income support (vs. welfare) is desirable (see rehabilitation therapy consultation below)
- Caregiver support and respite: if continuing to live with mother, ensure respite options. Provide mother and agency staff with guidance regarding role of "mental health" interventions

Psychosocial Treatment

- Behaviour management: functional behavioural assessment of anger profile and existing coping strategies, if any
- Counselling/Psychotherapy: role of social worker who is conducting family assessment and transitional case management
- Rehabilitation therapy: OT assessment to provide guidance regarding self-help, vocational goals, and social and recreational opportunities

Biomedical Treatment

- Medical treatment: follow-up monitoring as needed especially regarding health maintenance (including risk of obesity); oversee prescription of psychotropic drugs if recommended by psychiatry consultation
- Psychiatric treatment: consultation for differential diagnosis and treatment options related to working diagnosis of aggressive behaviour
- Residential and hospital treatment: may be needed if violent behaviour recurs as community treatment plan is being implemented

Prognosis

- Episodic course is predicted with reduced episodes through use of psychotropics, e.g., mood stabilizers and antipsychotic medications
- Social and vocational habilitative plan is extremely important—aim to see Ed working and living in a semi-supervised community residential option

Assessment for "John"

DC-LD Summary

Axis I Moderate intellectual disability

Axis II Unspecified etiology

Axis III Level D, sexually inappropriate behaviour

- Biologic factors: physically and sexually mature
- Psychologic factors: limited knowledge of sexuality issues and social-sexual expectations; rule out history of sexual abuse or peer group manipulation
- Social factors: parents extremely concerned and want to avoid criminal charges and further police involvement
- Developmental factors: special education class integrated in mainstream community school; expected to attend life skills program up to age 21

Health Problems

- Review recent medical assessments particularly any discussions of sexuality, peer group relationships, teasing, abuse

Resiliency Issues

- Review evidence of social and interpersonal relationships, including recreational outlets

Treatment-Management Plan for "John"

Developmental Services

- A place to live: maintain living arrangements with family
- Meaningful activities: maintain school program, establish level of instruction about human sexuality and interpersonal relationships
- Caregiver support and respite: provide guidance and support for parents as assessment and treatment plan are implemented; request parent-police case conference with clinician to explore details of complaint and arrangements for follow-up

Psychosocial Treatment

- Behaviour management: assess individual's level of social-sexual knowledge and provide individualized guidance (see counselling)
- Counselling/Psychotherapy: use results of psychosexual assessment to provide several sessions of sexuality education and guidance as related to insight into sexual behaviours

- Rehabilitation therapy: OT consultation to focus on provision of engaging options for leisure time

Biomedical Treatment

- Medical treatment: ensure primary care provider is fully aware of assessment results and psychosocial treatments being provided by clinic staff
- Psychiatric treatment: consultation available to clinic staff if there are concerns that the individual's difficulties go beyond those outlined above (e.g., paraphilias, gender identity problems, disorder of sexual preference)
- Residential/hospital treatment: not applicable in present circumstances

Prognosis

- Present "social crisis" can likely be fully resolved in 6–10 weekly visits to the clinic, if poor knowledge is main contributory factor
- Police, school, parents will monitor thereafter

Assessment for "Ted"

DC-LD Summary

Axis I Borderline intellectual functioning

Axis II Unspecified etiology

Axis III Level A, Asperger syndrome

- Biologic factors: review family history for evidence of mood and anxiety disorder
- Psychologic factors: review earlier assessment and school records to evaluate Ted's potential for a full or modified academic schedule at college
- Social factors: interview Ted to explore his level of anxiety regarding interpersonal relationships, mood problems, etc.
- Developmental factors: explore availability of special accommodations for academically and socially challenged students at community college (i.e., learning disability services)

Health Problems

- Review recent medical assessments particularly regarding evidence of anxiety, mood change, etc.

Resiliency Issues

- Review social-recreational pursuits, hobbies, spiritual beliefs

Treatment-Management Plan for "Ted"

Developmental Services

Note: Given borderline range of intellectual functioning, Ted may not qualify for developmental services; however, the college may make accommodations and mainstream health providers are available.

- A place to live: maintain current arrangement; or if college is in another community, explore its accommodation options
- Meaningful activities: review availability of special services at college for students with learning and social difficulties
- Caregiver support and respite: provide psychoeducation and support for mother; make recommendations for college "special services"

Psychosocial Treatment

- Behaviour management: not applicable presently, but may need anxiety management strategies in future
- Counselling/Psychotherapy: provide psychoeducation re: Asperger syndrome and mood disorder, and therapy regarding interpersonal issues
- Rehabilitation therapy: OT consultation as needed around challenges of leaving home and increasing level of independence; assess daily living skills

Biomedical Treatment

- Medical treatment: maintain contact with primary care provider for support
- Psychiatric treatment: consultation to assess depression, suicide risk, and potential for antidepressant medication
- Residential/hospital treatment: not applicable at present unless acute risk for self-harm

Prognosis

- Good prognosis for anxiety and mood that reflects anticipatory stress
- Rule out bipolar disorder in which case mood stabilizer and psychiatric follow-up is indicated

Assessment for "Sherri"

DC-LD Summary

Axis I Severe intellectual disability

Axis II Unknown etiology

Axis III Level D, self injurious behaviour (SIB)

- Biologic factors: rule out physical discomfort (e.g., wheelchair positioning, teeth, constipation, menstrual cramps, premenstrual dysphoria)
- Psychologic factors: functional behaviour assessment is needed to evaluate antecedents and consequences of SIB
- Social factors: explore relationships with family and agency caregivers including respite arrangements; rule out physical and sexual abuse or other "stressors"
- Developmental factors: explore availability of full-day or half-day program and access to weekend social and recreational options to increase meaningful activities

Health Problems

- Review results of annual health checks if available
- Review cerebral palsy status (muscle spasms, spasticity, joint limitations, inflammation, seating) from OT and PT perspective

Resiliency Issues

- Explore supportive relationships beyond family? Friends? Pets?
- Pursue "active" leisure pursuits—gym, pool, summer camps, educational trips

Treatment-Management for "Sherri"

Developmental Services

- A place to live: depending on review of family issues and available services, complete a transition plan for an alternative arrangement (e.g., group home or host family)
- Meaningful activities: ensure a full-day program and worthwhile weekend activities to increase meaningful activities and enhance resilience
- Caregiver support and respite: pending completion and implementation of transition plan, ensure support (including respite) for Sherri's mother. Family and day program need to be informed about results of functional behaviour assessment and approaches to eliminate or reduce episodic SIB

Psychosocial Treatment

- Behaviour management: therapist to complete functional behavioural assessment and evaluate approaches to both preventing recurrences and managing episodes in the least restrictive manner; evaluate assistive devices (e.g., helmet) if need be
- Counselling/Psychotherapy: only if family assessment reveals relevant issues
- Rehabilitation therapy: PT and OT participation in review of cerebral palsy status, seating, and design of leisure time activities

Biomedical Treatment

- Medical treatment: ensure review from perspective of discomfort prompting self-injurious behaviour and treat as needed (e.g., dental treatment, constipation, menstrual difficulties)
- Psychiatric treatment: only if functional behavioural assessment suggests mood or anxiety disorder or suitability of medication to modify threshold for self-injurious behaviour (e.g., baclofen, SSRI, vitamin B_6)
- Residential/hospital treatment: only if community approaches are not successful

Prognosis

- Results of functional behavioural assessment and availability of therapist to implement a behavioural plan and maintain monitoring
- Treatability of contributing medical factors (if detected)
- Resources for more recreational activities and respite for mother

Glossary

activities of daily living (ADL) – Daily self-care activities as a measurement of functional independence, for example, dressing, grooming, and feeding

adaptive behaviour – A set of daily living skills (dressing, toileting, etc.) and higher level communicative and social interaction skills used by people with disabilities to adjust to the demands of their environment

administrative prevalence – The number of cases of a disorder receiving service in a given population at a specific point in time

anencephaly – A serious defect in brain development associated with an incompletely formed skull and a variety of facial deformities. Incompatible with survival

applied behaviour analysis (ABA) – A scientifically validated approach to understanding and modifying behaviours by utilizing techniques and principles to bring meaningful and positive changes in behaviours

asphyxia – "Lack of oxygen," a possible cause of developmental disabilities when occurring around the time of delivery

attachment – The emotional connection or bond between child and caregiver that prevents an infant from aversive stress reactions in unfamiliar environments

Autism Diagnostic Observation Schedule – A standardized observation instrument that consists of structured and semi-structured activities (social, communicative, play) used in assessing children suspected of autism

behavioural phenotype – A specific behavioural profile seen in various genetic disorders, implying that the phenotype results from the underlying genetic abnormality

cerebral palsy (CP) – A loss or deficiency of motor control with involuntary spasms caused by permanent brain damage present at birth

challenging behaviour – Behaviour of such intensity, frequency, or duration that the physical safety of the person or others is likely to be placed in serious jeopardy; behaviour that is likely to seriously limit or deny access to the use of community resources

childhood disintegration disorder (CDD) – A pervasive developmental disorder characterized by late onset, before age 3, of developmental delays in language, social function, and motor skills

choreoathetosis – A movement disorder characterized by both chorea (involuntary purposeless movements) and athetosis (slow writhing movements)

congenital – Present at birth and either genetic or acquired in utero

Cornelia de Lange syndrome – A developmental disorder characterized by slow growth before and after birth, intellectual disability that is usually severe to profound, skeletal abnormalities involving the arms and hands, and distinctive facial features

counselling – Providing direction or advice as to a decision or course of action

CPAP (continuous positive airway pressure) – A type of assisted ventilation worn as a mask used in treatment of obstructive sleep apnea

deinstitutionalization – The relocation of persons with developmental disabilities from institutional settings to community residences

developmental disability – A condition characterized by significant limitations in intellectual functioning and in meeting normal standards of learning and productivity, with an onset in early life (prior to 18 years)

Down syndrome – A congenital disorder with particular physical features (e.g., small stature, up-slanting palprebal fissures, hypotonia) and mental characteristics (intellectual disability, predisposition to Alzheimer's disease, etc.) and associated with an extra chromosome (trisomy 21)

dual diagnosis – A developmental disability complicated by another mental disorder

dystonia – An abnormality of muscle tone that often leads to unusual posturing

eugenics – A social engineering philosophy to improve hereditary characteristics

euthanasia – The permitting or causing of death, usually in a person with a terminal illness or who is in a persistently vegetative state

fetal alcohol syndrome – A disorder with characteristic physical features (short stature, short palprebal fissures, smooth philtrum) and mental characteristics (intellectual or learning disability, predisposition to attentional problems) resulting from the teratogenic effects of maternal alcohol ingestion

fitness to stand – The ability for a defendant to understand the charges, participate in his or her own legal defense, and engage and follow in the court process

Flynn Effect – Substantial and long-sustained increase in intelligence test scores over the years measured in many parts of the world

Fragile X syndrome – A disorder with particular physical features (macrocephaly, large testicles) and mental characteristics (intellectual disability, autistic features) caused by a mutation of the X chromosome

functional behaviour assessment (FBA) – A problem-solving process for understanding the function and purpose of behaviour

gastroesophageal reflux disorder (GERD) – The regurgitation of stomach fluids and content back into the esophagus

hydrocephalus ("water on the brain") – An enlargement of the ventricles of the brain with an associated increase in the amount of cerebrospinal fluid. May be congenital or acquired

informed consent – The process by which a patient understands the nature of the proposed investigation or treatment and its anticipated outcome as well as the significant risks involved and alternative outcomes

instrumental activities of daily living (IADL) – Activities of daily living that are not necessary for fundamental functional independence (e.g., self-care) but allow one to live independently in the community (e.g., shopping, budgeting, domestic housework)

keratoconus – Conical protrusion of the centre of the cornea

Lennox-Gastaut syndrome – Severe intellectual disability, seizure, and spikes and slow waves on EEG; onset between age 2 and 6 years

mental capacity – The ability to perform mentally within the cognitive domain of thinking, reasoning, and problem-solving

mental competence – The ability to manage one's affairs, both personal and financial

mental disorder – A clinically significant behavioural or psychological syndrome or pattern that is typically associated with either a distressing symptom or an impairment of function

narcolepsy – A neurological disorder that results in both excessive daytime sleepiness and fragmented, poor quality nighttime sleep

neural tube – The brain and spinal cord in early fetal development

normalization – The philosophy and principle of providing persons with developmental disabilities the normal rhythms of life (daily, weekly, seasonally, etc.)

normative – Relating to or dealing with norms of average or common incidence in society

otoacoustic emissions – Sounds that are produced by healthy ears in response to outside sounds, used in screening hearing in children

pathogenesis – The mechanism by which the disease is caused

pathoplastic – Having the effect of altering characteristic features or symptoms

pervasive developmental disorder – Refers to a group of five developmental disorders characterized by delays in the development of multiple basic functions including language, socialization, and communication

phenylketonuria – A disorder with particular medical problems (microcephaly, epilepsy), intellectual disability and associated with a gene mutation causing an inability to metabolize phenylalanine. Preventable when recognized at birth by a diet with minimal amounts of phenylalanine

pica – The eating of dirt or non-edible items

Picture Exchange Communication System (PECS) – A form of augmentative alternative communication and typically used as an aid in communication for children with autism and other special needs

positive behavioural support (PBS) – Use of a system to understand what maintains an individual's challenging behaviour

Prader-Willi syndrome – A disorder with particular physical features (obesity, short stature) and mental characteristics (intellectual disability, obsessional patterns) due to an alteration of chromosome 15

psychopathology – Behavioural, emotional, personality, interpersonal, or somatic dysfunction in an individual

psychosis – A mental disorder that involves personality disintegration and loss of contact with reality including hallucinations, delusions, and positive and negative symptoms

psychotherapy – The treatment of mental or emotional problems by psychological means; talking therapeutic modalities, for example cognitive behaviour therapy

resilience – An ability to recover from or adjust to illness or trauma

Rett Syndrome – A disorder with particular physical features (microcephaly) and mental characteristics (autistic features, progressive loss of hand function) that progresses in young females and is associated with a mutation on the X chromosome

senescence – Increasing frailty and risk of disease and death the come with aging

sensory diet – A carefully designed, personalized activity plan that provides the sensory input a person needs to stay focused and organized throughout the day

sensory integration disorder – A disorder characterized by the inability to organize sensory information as it comes in through the senses

sleep apnea – Cessation of breathing during sleep

Smith-Magenis syndrome – A disorder with particular physical features (mid-facial hypoplasia, prominent jaw) and mental characteristics (intellectual disability, insomnia, pulling out one's nails) associated with a deletion of chromosome 17

spina bifida – A neural tube defect presenting with a failure of fusion of bones of the vertebral column and herniation of neural components

standardized test – A test that is administered and scored in a consistent, or "standard," manner

Stanford-Binet Intelligence Scale (5th edition) – A standardized test of general intelligence for persons ages 2–85+ years that yields verbal, non-verbal, and full-scale intelligence quotients with a mean of 100 versus a standard deviation of 15

stereotypic behaviours – Constantly repeated meaningless gestures or movements

Supports Intensity Scale – An instrument designed to directly measure the relative intensity of the support needs of a person with intellectual disabilities

syncope – A transient loss of consciousness due to inadequate blood flow to the brain

thimerosal – A mercury-containing preservative used in vaccine preparation

tics – Involuntary motor movements or repetitive twitching often in the face or upper trunk. Tourette syndrome is a neurological disorder characterized by severe motor and vocal tics

tuberous sclerosis – A disorder with particular physical features (skin lesions, lung and kidney cysts) and mental characteristics (intellectual disability, predisposition to autism), often with epilepsy and caused by a gene mutation on either chromosome 9 or 16

velocardiofacial syndrome – A disorder with particular physical features (cleft palate, congenital heart anomalies) and mental characteristics (intellectual disability, predisposition to psychosis) associated with a deletion of chromosome 22

Vineland Adaptive Behaviour Scale – A standardized measure of levels of adaptive behaviour often used in the diagnosis of an intellectual disability

Wechsler Adult Intelligence Scale (4th edition) – A standardized test of intelligence for persons ages 16–90 that yields a full-scale intelligence quotient, general ability index, and four index scores (verbal comprehension, perceptual reasoning, working memory, and processing speed)

West syndrome – A triad of infantile seizures, with a grossly disorganized EEG and developmental delay

Williams syndrome – A disorder with particular physical features (short stature, microcephaly) and mental characteristics (intellectual disability, sociability, anxiety) caused by a deletion of chromosome 7

About the Authors

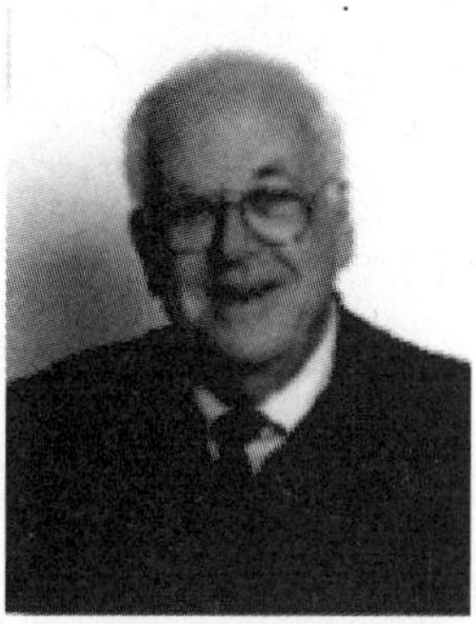

Bruce D. McCreary is Emeritus Professor of Psychiatry at Queen's University. He joined the Department of Psychiatry in 1968 and founded the Division of Developmental Disabilities in 1977. Dr. McCreary and colleagues provided mental health consulting services in the southeastern Ontario region; he retired from clinical practice in 2010 and presently contributes part-time to the division in teaching and scholarship. He is also a board member at Ongwanada, a local agency serving persons with developmental disabilities and their families. Ongwanada is formally affiliated with Queen's to foster teaching and research.

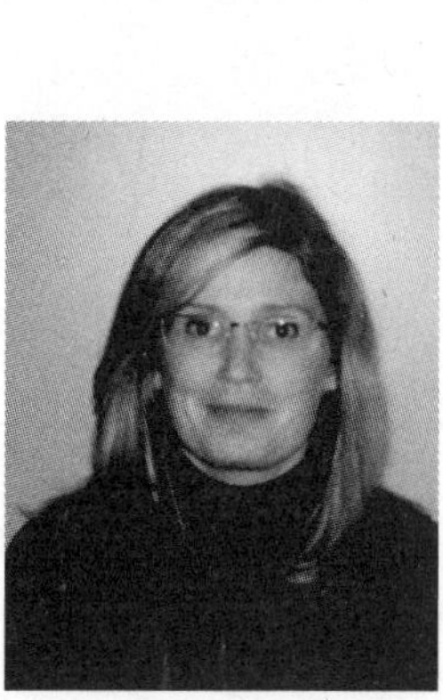

Jessica Jones, Associate Professor of Psychiatry and Psychology, is a clinical and forensic psychologist with the Queen's Department of Psychiatry, School of Medicine. She is the division chair of Developmental Disabilities and the clinical director of the Dual Diagnosis Program (DDCP), an interprofessional team providing services to children and adults with intellectual disabilities and mental health problems. Dr. Jones trained in the UK and has been working internationally with this population for over twenty years. Her particular interest is in forensic neuropsychiatry involving persons with dual diagnosis and autism spectrum disorders. Her research initiatives include challenging behaviour, risk assessment, Asperger's syndrome, and the unique clinical pathways and service system impact that offenders with disabilities have on the community.

INDEX

Queen's Policy Studies
Recent Publications

The Queen's Policy Studies Series is dedicated to the exploration of major public policy issues that confront governments and society in Canada and other nations.

Manuscript submission. We are pleased to consider new book proposals and manuscripts. Preliminary inquiries are welcome. A subvention is normally required for the publication of an academic book. Please direct questions or proposals to the Publications Unit by email at spspress@queensu.ca, or visit our website at: www.queensu.ca/sps/books, or contact us by phone at (613) 533-2192.

Our books are available from good bookstores everywhere, including the Queen's University bookstore (http://www.campusbookstore.com/). McGill-Queen's University Press is the exclusive world representative and distributor of books in the series. A full catalogue and ordering information may be found on their web site (**http://mqup.mcgill.ca/**).

For more information about new and backlist titles from Queen's Policy Studies, visit http://www.queensu.ca/sps/books.

School of Policy Studies

Building More Effective Labour-Management Relationships, Richard P. Chaykowski and Robert S. Hickey (eds.) 2013. ISBN 978-1-55339-306-1

Navigationg on the Titanic: Economic Growth, Energy, and the Failure of Governance, Bryne Purchase 2013. ISBN 978-1-55339-330-6

Measuring the Value of a Postsecondary Education, Ken Norrie and Mary Catharine Lennon (eds.) 2013. ISBN 978-1-55339-325-2

Immigration, Integration, and Inclusion in Ontario Cities, Caroline Andrew, John Biles, Meyer Burstein, Victoria M. Esses, and Erin Tolley (eds.) 2012. ISBN 978-1-55339-292-7

Diverse Nations, Diverse Responses: Approaches to Social Cohesion in Immigrant Societies, Paul Spoonley and Erin Tolley (eds.) 2012. ISBN 978-1-55339-309-2

Making EI Work: Research from the Mowat Centre Employment Insurance Task Force, Keith Banting and Jon Medow (eds.) 2012. ISBN 978-1-55339-323-8

Managing Immigration and Diversity in Canada: A Transatlantic Dialogue in the New Age of Migration, Dan Rodríguez-García (ed.) 2012. ISBN 978-1-55339-289-7

International Perspectives: Integration and Inclusion, James Frideres and John Biles (eds.) 2012. ISBN 978-1-55339-317-7

Dynamic Negotiations: Teacher Labour Relations in Canadian Elementary and Secondary Education, Sara Slinn and Arthur Sweetman (eds.) 2012. ISBN 978-1-55339-304-7

Where to from Here? Keeping Medicare Sustainable, Stephen Duckett 2012. ISBN 978-1-55339-318-4

International Migration in Uncertain Times, John Nieuwenhuysen, Howard Duncan, and Stine Neerup (eds.) 2012. ISBN 978-1-55339-308-5

Life After Forty: Official Languages Policy in Canada/Après quarante ans, les politiques de langue officielle au Canada, Jack Jedwab and Rodrigue Landry (eds.) 2011. ISBN 978-1-55339-279-8

From Innovation to Transformation: Moving up the Curve in Ontario Healthcare, Hon. Elinor Caplan, Dr. Tom Bigda-Peyton, Maia MacNiven, and Sandy Sheahan 2011. ISBN 978-1-55339-315-3

Academic Reform: Policy Options for Improving the Quality and Cost-Effectiveness of Undergraduate Education in Ontario, Ian D. Clark, David Trick, and Richard Van Loon 2011. ISBN 978-1-55339-310-8

Integration and Inclusion of Newcomers and Minorities across Canada, John Biles, Meyer Burstein, James Frideres, Erin Tolley, and Robert Vineberg (eds.) 2011. ISBN 978-1-55339-290-3

A New Synthesis of Public Administration: Serving in the 21st Century, Jocelyne Bourgon, 2011. ISBN 978-1-55339-312-2 (paper) 978-1-55339-313-9 (cloth)

Recreating Canada: Essays in Honour of Paul Weiler, Randall Morck (ed.), 2011. ISBN 978-1-55339-273-6

Data Data Everywhere: Access and Accountability? Colleen M. Flood (ed.), 2011. ISBN 978-1-55339-236-1

Making the Case: Using Case Studies for Teaching and Knowledge Management in Public Administration, Andrew Graham, 2011. ISBN 978-1-55339-302-3

Centre for International and Defence Policy

Afghanistan in the Balance: Counterinsurgency, Comprehensive Approach, and Political Order, Hans-Georg Ehrhart, Sven Bernhard Gareis, and Charles Pentland (eds.), 2012. ISBN 978-1-55339-353-5

Security Operations in the 21st Century: Canadian Perspectives on the Comprehensive Approach, Michael Rostek and Peter Gizewski (eds.), 2011. ISBN 978-1-55339-351-1

Institute of Intergovernmental Relations

Canada and the Crown: Essays on Constitutional Monarchy, D. Michael Jackson and Philippe Lagassé (eds.), 2013. ISBN 978-1-55339-204-0

Paradigm Freeze: Why It Is So Hard to Reform Health-Care Policy in Canada, Harvey Lazar, John N. Lavis, Pierre-Gerlier Forest, and John Church (eds.), 2013. ISBN 978-1-55339-324-5

Canada: The State of the Federation 2010, Matthew Medelsohn, Joshua Hjartarson, and James Pearce (eds.), 2013. ISBN 978-1-55339-200-2

The Democratic Dilemma: Reforming Canada's Supreme Court, Nadia Verrelli (ed.), 2013. ISBN 978-1-55339-203-3

The Evolving Canadian Crown, Jennifer Smith and D. Michael Jackson (eds.), 2011. ISBN 978-1-55339-202-6

The Federal Idea: Essays in Honour of Ronald L. Watts, Thomas J. Courchene, John R. Allan, Christian Leuprecht, and Nadia Verrelli (eds.), 2011. ISBN 978-1-55339-198-2 (paper) 978-1-55339-199-9 (cloth)

The Democratic Dilemma: Reforming the Canadian Senate, Jennifer Smith (ed.), 2009. ISBN 978-1-55339-190-6